960

Healer's Handbook

Healer's Handbook

A Holistic Guide to Wellness in the New Age

Patricia Telesco

SAMUEL WEISER, INC.

York Beach, Maine

First published in 1997 by
Samuel Weiser, Inc.
P. O. Box 612
York Beach, ME 03910-0612

Library of Congress Cataloging-in-Publication Data

Telesco, Patricia.
    Healer's handbook : a holistic guide to wellness in the new
age / Patricia Telesco.
        p.   cm.
    Includes bibliographical references and index.
    ISBN 1-57863-018-5 (alk. paper)
    1. Alternative medicine. 2. Holistic medicine. I. Title.
R733.T45   1997
615.5—dc21   97-17739
                                                    CIP

MG

Typeset in 11 point New Baskerville

Cover art is "The Uprising" copyright © 1997 by Norbert Lösche.
Used by permission. Walter Holl Agency, Germany.

Printed in the United States of America

04 03 02 01 00 99 98 97
10 9 8 7 6 5 4 3 2 1

The paper used in this publication meets the minimum
requirements of the American National Standard for Permanence
of Paper for Printed Library Materials Z39.48-1984.

TABLE OF CONTENTS

TABLES

CREDITS

Quoted material introducing text comes from the following sources:

Page xi: Introduction: Samuel Johnson, *New Dictionary of Thoughts,* Tyson Edwards, ed.(New York: Standard Book Company, 1936), p. 247.

Page 1: Manly P. Hall, *Secret Teachings of All Ages* (Los Angeles, CA: Philosophical Research Society, 1977), p. 178.

Page 24: Diodorus Siculus, in *New Dictionary of Thoughts,* Tyson Edwards, ed.(New York: Standard Book Company, 1936), p. 382.

Page 47: Paracelsus, *The Paragranum,* translation by Franz Hartmann, in Manly P. Hall, *Secret Teachings of All Ages* (Los Angeles, CA: Philosophical Research Society, 1977), p. 109.

Page 49: Rollo May, *Man's Search for Himself* (New York: New American Library, 1953), p. 94.

Page 59: John Milton, *Paradise Lost,* Book IV, lines 644–647.

Page 72: Eliphas Levi, *History of Magic* (York Beach, ME: Samuel Weiser, 1970; London: Rider, 1969), p. 256.

Page 95: John Greenleaf Whittier, "Raphael," Stanza 16.

Page 108: Francois, Duc de Rochefoucauld, Maxim 403, in *New Dictionary of Thoughts,* Tyson Edwards, ed. (New York: Standard Book Company, 1936), p. 201.

Page 119: Isaiah 54:11, 12. Biblical quotes from King James version of The Holy Bible (New York: Harper & Brothers, n.d.).

Page 132: Henry Wadsworth Longfellow, "Keramos."

Page 152: Fritjof Capra, *The Tao of Physics* (Boston: Shambhala, 1975), p. 69.

Page 167: Robinson Jeffers, from "Boats in a Fog," in *Familiar Quotations,* John Bartlett (Boston: Little Brown, 1938).

Page 178: William Blake, "Auguries of Innocence," in *The Oxford Dictionary of Quotations,* 2nd ed. (London: Oxford University Press, 1955), p. 73.

Page 184: Henry David Thoreau, "Higher Laws" in *Walden, The Portable Thoreau,* Carl Bode, ed. (London: Penguin, 1977), p. 468.

Page 200: Dr. Wallace MacNaughton, Brett Bravo, *Crystal Healing Secrets* (New York: Warner Books, 1988), p. 211.

Page 210: Quintilian, *Institutiones Oratoriae,* in *New Dictionary of Thoughts,* Tyson Edwards, ed.(New York: Standard Book Company, 1936), p. 241.

Page 219: William Shakespeare, *King Henry VI,* Part II, III, 31.

Page 235: Jeannine Parvati Baker, from an article titled "Hands that Heal." Used by permission.

Page 245: Maharishi Mahesh Yogi, in Bodo Baginski, *Reiki* (Los Angeles, CA: Life Rhythm Publications, 1988).

Page 252: William Cowper, *The Task:* Book VI, *The Winter Walk at Noon,* l.I.

FOREWORD

Alternative medicine has grown tremendously in both its knowledge and techniques in recent years. Consequently, the information contained herein is by no means complete. The instructions provided are reasonably safe for anyone to try. Nonetheless, no book can (or should) supercede formalized training in some of these fields, especially those like midwifery, where one's skill may literally become the deciding factor in a life-or-death situation.

Neither the author nor the publisher can warrant or guarantee any results from the methods presented here. While ancient in origins, alternative medicine in its modern rebirth is still in its infancy, and should be treated with appropriate caution. Similarly, in no way should the information or instructions presented here be considered a replacement for modern medicine.

There are many additional alternative paths to wellness, and many variations or "schools" other than those explored in this book. It would take several volumes to cover all aspects of New Age healthcare. Therefore, I have tried to provide "snapshots" of a few with which I am more personally familiar. Some techniques have been left out of this "photo album." Any such exclusions should not be taken as a sign that a particular methodology is ineffective or unethical. It was simply a matter of space and my own inability to responsibly report on those methods.

Finally, to both healers and their patients, I wish you well. It's not easy being on either side of healing process, but it is an experience you're not likely to forget. For a few brief moments, two people stand outside of time and space for the sole purpose of finding that elusive quality known as wholeness. When their efforts work, no matter the technique, it is truly a miracle for which one should rejoice and give thanks.

INTRODUCTION

To preserve health is a moral and religious
duty, for health is the basis of all social
virtues.
—Samuel Johnson

Those with the ability to make us feel better—emotionally, physically, or spiritually—have always been an important cornerstone in any community. Exactly who were these people? One was an ancient village shaman, another a medieval monk; some were rural cunning folk, others were caring mothers, and some were trained physicians. No matter their title, however, people around the world, down through history, have found ways to reach out and help others reclaim wholeness. This is a special heritage, and one which the New Age movement has done much to reclaim.

This modern spiritual awakening is accompanied by the recognition of an age-old trinity central to well-being: the unity of body, mind, and soul. We all yearn for, and desperately need, this balance. In answer to this need, spiritually-centered healing approaches have emerged out of the New Age vogue. With them come many questions from people who want to get involved in these arts, and people who want to try different techniques for personal wellness.

Several of these questions recur regularly. From where are these "new" health approaches coming? Are they viable? How do you learn them? The answer to the second question must come from your own heart. The answer to the third can be found in this book.

In answer to the first query, the phrase "there is nothing new under the Sun" comes to mind. Many New Age (or "alternative") medicines have origins that are hundreds, if not thousands, of years old. In truth, hands-on healing methods whisper of long-forgotten moments in human existence when our spiritual nature was not separate from everyday life; times when metaphysical beliefs played an important role in shaping our thoughts and actions; times when nature was our pharmacy and our wits kept us alive.

A prime illustration here is the use of crystals in auric work. Many ancient cultures revered stones as magical, and ascribed specific qualities to nearly every gem unearthed. The Chinese used jade as a protective amulet; Germans carried beryl to safeguard themselves from slothfulness; and the Babylonians believed hematite had the ability to charm others. The people employing these stones were not always experts, and many did not regard the applications as magical. Instead, people felt that this power was an accessible part of nature provided by the gods for anyone's use, if they could but learn how.

For example, since amber portrayed the ability to ensnare insects, early people thought it equally valuable for capturing maladies! So, when a modern practitioner of auric healing chooses to use amber placed on or near an inflicted area as part of a treatment, this is nothing new. Instead, it is a venerable old custom being reborn with a slightly different focus.

Healer's Handbook was written with this rich birthright in mind. While training is important to metaphysical healing, the world of healing is not an exclusive club that only a few select people may enter. By combining a heartfelt desire and spiritual sensitivity with education, you can begin mobilizing your full healing potential.

Healer's Handbook describes ways to discern if you have a natural gift or propensity for the healing arts. If you do, then it helps you determine exactly what aspect(s) or skills to pursue. It shares the history of several metaphysical methods, portrays ancient and modern techniques, shares personal accounts, and tells you about the people who shaped those systems. It also provides some "hands-on" exercises that can improve your skill and confidence. In instances where these pages speak of more schooled abilities (like Reiki or midwifery), contact addresses or phone numbers are provided for further information.

Healer's Handbook also takes an honest look at alternative medicines: their benefits, scope, and limitations. Many people have justifiable concerns and a healthy dose of skepticism about unfamiliar healing methods. Thus, books like this help provide basic information to use as a guideline when considering New Age techniques for personal care.

Beyond all this, *Healer's Handbook* seeks to undo some of the negative connotations that surround natural and metaphysical healing techniques. There is nothing absurd or silly about believing that wellness depends partially on spirit-related matters. I truly believe it has been the modern sequestration of the spiritual and sacred that has led to much of our dis-ease. Thus, even if these methods are only learned and applied as an adjunct to commonly accepted medical practices to heal the soul, the effort is more than worthwhile.

Those who wish to enter the practice of alternative medicine today have a difficult task ahead of them. The world is hurting; people are hurting. It takes tremendous love and personal commitment to reach out and begin treating those wounds. Yet, it can happen. Let us join together in peace and begin transforming our reality. Through small acts of healing, performed one at a time, healers can love this world into wholeness. Let it begin today with you.

Part 1

A Healer's Role, Rights, and Responsibilities

*And these kindly folk are believed to have
held as their purpose of existence the healing
of the sick in mind, soul, and body.*
—Manly Palmer Hall
regarding the Essenes

The Human Factor: Me, a Healer?

Healers must be the world's greatest lovers,
for you must love something to make it whole.
—The LoreSinger

ALTERNATIVE MEDICINE REDIRECTS THE FOCUS OF healing to the whole person—thus the modern phrase "holistic." In the healing process, an individual becomes an outlet for Universal Energy, and the technique used equates to an extension cord for transmitting that energy. So in effect, the central skill for any good healer is the ability to connect with that universal socket—an ability that virtually any spiritually aware person can learn. No matter who you are or what your outlook may be, if you have a sincere desire to do it, you can have the capacity to become the conduit for some type of hands-on healing.

Actually, once your studies begin, you may discover a spiritual knack that has been with you all along, disguised in a different form. Perhaps you have always been a caregiver, a motherly type, someone fascinated by medicine, someone who loves working the land. Perhaps you just hate to see anyone or anything suffer.

No matter your personal scenario, alternative medicine offers much to both the practitioner and the patient. For an introvert, for example, a newly acquired knowledge or ability in the healing arts may help overcome social awkwardness. Shy people quickly see how valuable their listening skills are as part of the healer's "black bag." Similarly, extroverts are people who have been the proverbial cheerleaders and motivators all their lives. Now they can begin using that positive energy to manifest emotional and physical wellness through their efforts.

HOW DO I KNOW FOR SURE?

How do you know if learning and practicing alternative healing methods is "right" for you? This is a fundamental question because of the responsibility involved, and the need to be careful about the way you use healing energy. For example, I don't suggest that everyone reading the chapter on touch therapy rush right out and try to "lay hands" on the sick. Instead, I advise careful consideration of your motivations, spiritual abilities, areas of knowledge, and reasons for wanting to work in this field. Frequently, the best answer is found during those quiet moments of prayer or meditation between you, yourself, and the divine.

This question is also difficult because assurance comes in different forms for different people. Generally speaking, many healers contacted for this effort relate what I call the "Aha!" syndrome. In effect, one day, a flicker of confidence and awareness suddenly ignited in their spirit. The cause of that initial spark varied, but it was unquenchable and empowering. If such a moment hasn't come for you yet, try asking yourself these questions:

Does it seem as if you have always been helping or healing in some way or another? Many healers tell me that, as children, they put bandaids on their toys or pets, tried to comfort other crying children, or were always fixing things. As adults, they found people coming to them regularly for similar services—a solid shoulder to lean on or someone to "make it better"—even though they never openly revealed any propensity for the healing arts.

Have you encountered repeated unusual circumstances that cause you to "take charge" as a healer? The universe is not always subtle in its workings. If, for example, you find yourself alone on a regular basis with friends who have headaches and no aspirin, this may be a hint. Once or twice can be counted as coincidence, but when cycles repeat themselves in life, it's usually for a good reason. Stop and listen to the small voice of Spirit in that situation; then let your heart guide you.

To balance this statement, be careful about over-spiritualizing the mundane. Someone can have a kink in their neck because they sat in a funny position on the couch, not because you're supposed to jump in with aid! Remain sensitive and open to those messages, lessons, or the lack thereof that every moment of living offers.

Have you had dreams or visions in which you've received reasonable instructions in the healing arts? In ancient China, Babylon, and Egypt, priests and leaders often sequestered themselves in temples to receive dreams or visions. A number of these dream oracles concerned themselves with matters of health. So there is a historical precedent for healing as a visionary art. One of the individuals interviewed later in this chapter received their instructions in this manner. I must caution, however, that such instances are uncommon.

Psychologists, including Sigmund Freud and C. G. Jung, indicate that dreams can reveal personal struggles or insights of which we are unaware in waking hours. Even so, we often find it difficult to take them seriously. The modern mind regards dreams mostly as flights of fancy. I believe the attitude that regards dream interpretation as an obsolete and quaint custom may be partially blamed for the decrease in visionary teachings today.

It is easy to mistake the symbolism of dreams: hence the caution to use rationality and reasonableness in your consideration of them. If you envision peanut butter and jelly as a cure for cancer, perhaps there is some medical evidence that could support your theory. However, I suspect this example was driven more by a craving than a true spiritual experience.

In either case, I suggest keeping a log of your dreams so you can review them regularly. They may reveal important ideas or trends that you've missed. Whether or not you finally choose to involve yourself in healing, you are a divine creature with tremendous potential. Don't overlook any opportunity to hone your spiritual nature.

Have you met another talented healer who has taken interest in teaching you? There is an old saying about teachers coming along when you really need them, not necessarily when you want them. If someone has taken a special interest in you, it's probably for a very good reason. They see potential in you, like a seed just waiting to sprout.

The question in this case is, do you want to pursue this specific direction? If so, then welcome their offer of education and insights. If not, at least consider the fact that one healing avenue was open to you. That may mean others are as well. Don't close opportunity's door. Look at this as a chance to examine your feelings about alternative medicine and possible outlets for any talents you possess.

Did you ever think that you might have been involved in healing in another life? Sometimes our souls remember things that we consciously do not. This spiritual diary guides us from our earliest youth onward toward something familiar and comfortable. Having been a healer in a past life does not require a repeat performance in this one. However, if you have felt a perplexing urge or tendency, this may be one explanation. Past-life experiences can provide foundational skill sets to those who feel they should walk this path again.

Do you have the ability to discern auric energy without really trying through any one of your senses? Not an absolute necessity, but very helpful. Discernment of auric energy has many other applications besides healing. So in and of itself, this isn't an absolute indicator. When combined with other affirmative answers to the questions on this list, however, this makes a pretty strong case.

Can you instinctively tell when someone is out of sorts and sometimes even what's wrong with another person without being given any information? At first, this ability seems miraculous in a world where only doctors, tests, and X-ray machines reveal the source of sickness. Yet, if you believe in the individual nature of energy and the way physical conditions affect that energy, then logic dictates that sensing those energy changes is possible. This is especially true of empathic people, or those whose senses have been trained to spot clues. For such individuals, indicators can come through the aura, a scent, a sound, an odd feeling, or body language, to name just a few.

In an effort to confirm these flashes of intuition, ask the person involved if the hunch is true. Keep a detailed record of your successes and failures. Accurate observations 70 percent of the time indicate that either you have this ability or you are an incredibly lucky guesser. It is up to you to decide which conclusion is correct.

Have you always known that you wanted to help others through healing and instinctively understood what form worked best for you? Another somewhat rare occurrence, but by no means impossible. There are some individuals who simply accept their roles with nonchalant poise and dignity. If you are among this number, count yourself fortunate and move forward with your training.

DISCOVERING HEALING TALENTS by Loba Hardin[1]

There seem to be two elements to discovering one's path in healing as a service to others and this planet. The first is being truly "called," fated, and equipped for service in spite of personal uncertainties. Besides the ecstacy it engenders, there is a painful intensity attending awareness, empathy, clairvoyance and precognition that scares many people away from their desired path, or natural healing abilities. The second element is one's full acceptance of the responsibilities of a healer. In essence, learning healing arts requires a personal contract with the Greater Self, one's soul, with the Earth and Spirit.

For Jesse Wolf Hardin[2] the vocation for healing was loud and unimpeachable. The voice within made it difficult to sleep—spiritual eyes made it impossible not to see the suffering of others—spiritual vision made it hard not to exceed personal limits set by society. For him, the message of need and an empowering drive came through the voices of the birds, on the wind, and through missives unscrolled by columns of ants on their way to the nest.

Turned off by church experiences, he never called this motivational energy "god," but simply called it "magic"—the great mystery that one could always feel was the will of Gaia, and thus of all Creation, gently leading. This voice bid him to try various paths from Pow-Wows to the Nordic tradition. Finally, he turned away from all these and listened to Spirit directly. Here he discovered that all healers and visionaries access the same reservoir of power and direction.

As with most who are drawn to healing arts, Wolf had to struggle to accommodate reality, education, dogma, financial pressures, government regulation and a culture of denial with integrity. There are forever those who cling to comfort and certainty

---

[1]Loba G. Hardin, The Earthen Spirituality Project. Used by permission.
[2]For more information about Jesse Wolf Hardin, see chapter 8, "Earthly Realms," page 158, and bibliography for books available.

at all costs—who are unwilling to see, feel and experience the power of healing and balance. Because of this, Wolf believes that one can be sure of their healing abilities, sure of their chosen paths toward wellness, at the point when they realize, in the face of every difficulty, that they can do nothing else . . . when the only choices they can make are difficult, but right . . . when they "dare to love so much."

One final note: the eight questions given above were assembled by comparing consistent trends in interviews with people involved in alternative medicine. Nonetheless, they are not hard and fast rules. Even if all of your answers to all the questions were negative, don't let that dissuade a sincere desire. The marvelous part about New Age ideology is recognizing the uniqueness of the human soul and its capacity to grow in unexpected and profound ways. If your spirit yearns for the growth and discipline that practicing the healing arts provides, then move bravely ahead with your heartfelt assurance as a guide.

WHY ME?

Almost everyone involved in alternative medicine has asked themselves these questions at least once along the way. Isn't there someone else more suited to this job? Why me?

The favorite reply from the universe usually consists of a simple phrase: "Because you said, 'yes.'" Somewhere along the line, the Spirit sent out a message of need to which you responded. It sounds too simple, you say? Instinctive, intuitive things usually are exactly that!

Breaching the "why me?" barrier is the most arduous task. Most people find it difficult to believe that they can function as a channel to help themselves and others. Yet, if we truly believe in the life-energy that permeates all living things, this possibility seems less miraculous and more natural, which is how it should seem.

Right-brain thinking is what makes the entire process seem as if it should be more complex. Where's the flash and the fanfare? Where's the mysterious encounter with divine voices and powers? Those experiences, while nice to bolster one's confidence, are few and far between. Just as a patient must trust the healer for aid, healers-in-training must trust their gut instincts, knowledge and spiritual gifts for guidance. They must also rely on the universe to know what's best.

Morgana's Story [3]

Everything happens when it's supposed to . . . and my desire to learn about healing started around 1990, six years after being told by a psychic that I had a natural talent. Why so long? I didn't really accept my potential or power . . . the self confidence wasn't there. I had to grow and accept that aspect of myself, which I now recognize as an undeniable part of my soul.

The very first experience with my own healing ability came through a friend. He had a singing engagement and his throat was quite sore. I awkwardly offered to help, then began concentrating intensely, hoping I was proceeding correctly. There was nothing overly spectacular about the whole process. I just placed my hand near his throat to draw out the problem. Tom felt this manifest physically as a tingling in the larynx, then pronounced that his throat felt "different" and better.

That was my debut, in all its glorious simplicity.

Morgana's story illustrates many important points, the greatest of which is that healing can be potent and produc-

---

[3]Used by permission. See chapter 3, "Auric Cleansing and Balancing," page 72.

tive without Hollywood effects. It also shows how much confidence it takes to begin walking down the healer's path. Mind you, there is nothing wrong with having some uncertainties and fears. Both keep us honest with ourselves and others.

A healthy dose of skepticism also checks conceit. There is a lot of personal culpability in this service-oriented skill. Anything that maintains the delicate balance between assurance and arrogance may be regarded as a "good thing."

The only time to really worry about doubts is when they begin to make you ineffectual. Fear can be immobilizing, and can result in a terrible waste of talent. If you ever feel yourself reaching this point, take time off to get a fresh perspective. Seek out other healers for council and support. Read the latest books on your area of expertise. Meditate, eat healthy foods, and get some decent rest. Renewing the well of self lets you return to your tasks refreshed, revitalized, and reassured.

LEVELS OF COMMITMENT

Generally speaking, I recommend that people pursue one specific type of healing path for a minimum of one year as a part-time "hobby," if you will (unless it's a schooled technique). This allows you to be certain you've chosen the right branch of the tree for your personality. It also allows you to decide how deeply involved in the healing arts you wish to become.

People with healing knowledge do not necessarily have to work "full-time" at their art. Don't feel all other aspects of your normal life have to come to a screeching halt the minute you learn a healing skill. After this trial period, you can decide the level of commitment that's right for your circumstances and spirit.

Some people may find they want to pursue a career in alternative medicine. To do this, you will probably have to obtain proper certification according to state and federal mandates. Check the laws in your region and review the Yellow Pages to see if anyone in your area may be able to offer advice on how to proceed on this issue. Alternatively, use the contact addresses or phone numbers in the appropriate section of this book for more information.

Other individuals may discover that, while the healing arts are helpful to them, they aren't something they want to embrace as a full-time job. There is nothing wrong with this. After all, if we were all doctors, who would pave the streets? Individuals must trust their hearts to know how best to proceed. If you've chosen what I consider "on call" healing, use your new-found insight and knowledge as needs arise (or when you feel strongly led). Also, use your experience to teach others desirous of learning the healing arts. In the process, you will be helping full-time healers by filling in the gaps that come from there being so many needy people and only twenty-four hours in a day!

Marian's Personal Story[4]

When I first got involved in the New Age movement, I had no idea that I would ever be involved in healing arts. Yet, when I began reaching deeper states of meditation, the image of a man came to me again and again. His voice echoed in my mind with information on how to relieve pain. The methods seemed simple enough and very symbolic in nature. Yet, no one ever told me what this might mean.

Then, one weekend after about a year of these visions appearing regularly, I was out camping with some friends. One of the men in our group had an argument with gravity and twisted his

---

[4]Used by permission.

ankle. He came limping toward the fire and sat down with a sad face, thinking his entire weekend was ruined.

Before I had a chance to think about what I was saying, the words, "I think I can help if you'll let me try," came rolling out of my mouth. I swear, to this day, I don't know how or why I suddenly felt it was time; but there it was. Now I was committed to action!

When he said "yes," I stumbled through a brief personal meditation and began the auric balancing and massage combination that I'd seen in my meditations. At first, it felt odd and awkward, but within a few minutes the energy just flowed. The palms of my hands got warm and tingly. I knew I was becoming a conduit for divine power, so I relaxed and really tried to focus that energy.

I guided my hands over the injured area and could actually feel the itchy spot in his aura where the twisted muscle occurred. Using visualization and hand movements, I symbolically smoothed out the region. Much to my amazement (and, I suspect, to his), he felt much better afterward. My fears were transformed by that experience into trust, confidence, and a healthy bit of relief. I wasn't crazy after all!

From that day forward, I knew I would be doing more work of this nature from time to time. For one thing, I was now more willing to offer aid when a need evidenced itself. Also, as the years wore on, I found myself teaching others the simple techniques that started that day, and those people have gone on to do likewise. Through sharing our successful approaches, healing has become like a splashing fountain that touches many people daily, and sometimes we're not even aware that we've touched them.

SIX TYPES OF HEALING APTITUDES

Not everyone who studies alternative healing methods will work "miracles." Historically speaking, that job was usually left to a few wise masters like Jeshua ben Joseph, Ghandi, and Mother Teresa. Jeshua healed people's bodies, Ghandi their minds and spirits, and Mother Teresa ministered to both body and soul. These three people demonstrate the pinnacle of what a healing vocation can become.

However, no mountain is complete without the soil that forms its foundations. Similarly, healthcare is not complete without the aid of many people with various abilities, each of which is important. Just because you can't make a lame person walk in minutes doesn't mean your service is ineffectual. You may have provided this sufferer with their first taste of glorious relief. That is where everything begins—with rekindled hope.

Thus, I encourage you to read this section very carefully and try to find yourself herein. As you do, be fully aware that no type of healing proficiency is "better" than any other. These are just different talents and approaches suited to the uniqueness of individuals. Bear in mind also that the exact way each of these types manifests itself will differ according to the technique applied to achieve the goal, and that one person may exhibit more than one type.

I also urge caution in what gets categorized as a metaphysically based healing method. There is no rule that says an adept surgeon cannot be exercising a spiritual talent. Conversely, nothing says that all herbalists are spiritually inclined. Thus, what determines this factor is not the medium, but the individual's perspective toward the work.

Type 1: Bringing Sleep

Our bodies and minds can not work effectively when we are tired. Physicians have always recommended that their patients "get plenty of rest." Patients, however, are not always cooperative. This is where someone gifted in sleep aids comes in very handy. Through their knowledge and talent, they can help a stubborn or terribly uncomfortable person get necessary rest. This then helps the body work more efficiently and speeds the healing process.

Various techniques can be used here with equally impressive effect. An herbalist may make a special tea blend or recommend specific herbal supplements to the diet. A massage therapist soothes the muscles while playing relaxing tapes in the background. Someone who has strong telepathic abilities may connect with the patient's mind and give it a gentle nudge toward sleep. Each approach is perfectly valid.

Some healers who work in this area have a potpourri of spiritual gifts that get combined to improve overall results: for example, providing an herbal tea first, followed by a touch therapy session that includes a guided meditation. No matter the approach, the healer's goal is to teach the patient the art of relaxation for health.

While coaxing is sometimes necessary for obstinate types who refuse to sit down, this will do little good over the long haul. Healers must also educate people to take care of the temple of their souls; the body. Similarly, they must always take care that their actions do not violate another's free will. If someone *asks* for help, it may be given, but it should never be forced.

Type 2: Pain Relief

This works hand in hand with any number of other abilities listed here. Just as sleep helps the body accept spiritual healing efforts more readily, so does the abatement of pain. Pain causes tension throughout the body. For example, if your neck gets stiff, you often experience a headache, too. This is stress, discomfort, and dis-ease as manifested through the human neural web. Pain also decreases concentration and personal energy.

So, pain relief (even temporary) is a vital part of the healing equation. Those gifted in this area usually have highly attuned senses. When they meet someone with an active problem, the problem evidences itself through those senses. For example, a pain reliever who meets someone with knee trouble may notice that problem through an ache or itch around his or her own knee. Or perhaps he or she will see an auric abnormality in that area. In either case, knowing the exact location of pain helps the pain reliever guide and direct energy more accurately.

In this illustration, an herbalist could prepare a special liniment with plants picked during a waning Moon to symbolically encourage "shrinking" pain. He or she might also show a patient how to apply the liniment for best results. As with Marian's story earlier in this chapter, the auric balancer moves clean, white light into the auric field, realigning the patient's energy, thereby improving overall well-being. Someone knowledgeable about pressure points may use that awareness during massage to redirect pain, allowing healing energy to flow unhindered.

Again, you can see the frequency of using combined techniques. While most healers have one specialty, many quickly discover the advantages to being versed in different areas. Because they already have the basic skill sets and knowledge necessary, learning the rudiments of alternative techniques is not terribly difficult. Actually, the exploration readily unearths latent symbiotic abilities. For example, an auric balancer may discover tremendous aptitude for massage. Or, a person enacting guided meditations might detect a talent for past-life regressions. The key in all cases is remaining open and aware of yourself, your patient, and the sacred energies that link you together.

Type 3: Physical Manifestation

The physical manifestor produces medically verifiable results in varying degrees. The treatment by an herbalist often brings some relief to a cold in a fairly short time, for example. A holistician treats more serious maladies with long-term recommendations that aid recuperation and rejuvenation. A physical therapist can give nearly immediate relief from pain, if only temporarily.

Profound, immediate physical manifestations sometimes come under the heading of "miracles" because it outwardly appears that spectacular changes have occurred. The reason for this is threefold: the patient's trust, the healer's level of expertise, and the overall effectiveness of the technique for the manifested problem. Nonetheless, "miraculous" healings are rare because of the apprehension surrounding New Age approaches. Negative press has produced nervous healers and cynical patients. When we consider the last time a miracle healer walked this Earth and the way he was received, their misgivings seem sensible.

Thus, only a few who have a knack for physical manifestation will experience dramatic results. Yet, subtle workings shouldn't be underestimated in their importance. Physical manifestation over time is just as necessary. Actually, some conditions need slow, gentle care for the most effective outcomes.

It is because of this unique balance that I caution physical manifestors against pushing for too much progress too soon. The hardest part of having this talent is not succumbing to the "faster is better" ideology. It is normal to be enthusiastic when you see corroborated results for your efforts, but Mother Nature still needs to have her way.

This lesson holds true for all healing arts and all types of healing abilities. We must always remind ourselves that universal laws do not stop or take detours when healing occurs. This means we must try to follow the voices of spirit and reason down the path to wholeness, and not succumb to our own enthusiasm.

Physical manifestors are like pain relievers in that they may have spiritual cues that help them in their work. Exactly what these cues are varies for each person. Additionally, these people (except faith healers) are often professionally trained in their field, allowing them to extend reliable knowledge with a helping hand.

In a February 1995 edition of the *Wall Street Journal,* rolphing, myotherapy, naturopathy, feldenkrais, midwifery, osteopathy and massage therapy were all named as having gained recognition from the insurance industry as coverable expenses. Many practicing these techniques linger near the edge of New Age ideology, while others adopt it wholeheartedly. In other words, metaphysical healing is coming of age. Physical manifestors are an integral part of creating this new form of health coverage because their techniques are documentable, productive, and cost effective.

Type 4: Emotional Care-Givers

The ultimate support unit, care-givers are universal "mommies." These people have the ability to make us feel better just by being around. They bolster our confidence, show pride in our accomplishments, bring us soup or call when we're sick, and always stand ready with hugs, no matter the reason.

Emotional care-givers are a very important piece in the puzzle of healing. They fill in a lot of the little gaps left by other methodologies. For while herbalists can recommend a good tea for the flu, they usually won't stop by to hold your hand. Physical manifestors may only work with their patients a certain number of hours a week, in a clinical environment. The care-giver, however, steps into this void gladly and often without being asked.

These are people who need to wear a pin that says: "Stop me before I volunteer again." Care-givers are very generous with their energy, sometimes to a fault. They can easily overextend themselves because there are so many needy people. It is very difficult for the care-giver to say no. In fact, about the only way to slow down a care-giver is by another care-giver meeting them head-on!

With this in mind, make every effort not to take advantage of the care-givers in your life. Their zealous service makes it tempting to ask for aid, even in moments when you could get along on your own. At these junctures, remember the generous spirit you're dealing with and consider if you *really* need help. There may be someone else who could benefit far more from the care-giver's assistance. For that matter, they may need a break from their toils.

Similarly, if you find yourself in this category, I urge caution with your personal health and well-being. Nothing productive will get done if you are ill or out of sorts. It takes a tremendous amount of compassion to be an effective care-giver, and this type of energy does not flow well through a neglected vessel. So, remember to give back a little of that special attention to yourself once in a while.

Because care-givers serve the lonely, shut-ins, invalids, and others who feel somehow secluded because of their malady, listening makes up a good portion of this type of healing. It is one of the hardest talents to develop and perfect. Fortunately, many care-givers have a natural knack with impartial listening skills. They allow free-flowing conversation where convalescents can openly and honestly discuss their feelings without fear of judgment. By being proactive listeners, care-givers help people rediscover their own inner strength, insight, and vision.

Care-givers have a tremendous creative force behind them. They stimulate change, have abundant ideas, motivate stagnant energy, and always supply alternative perspectives. Thus, care-givers provide healing to the hearts and spirits of others through their sensitive labors.

Type 5: Spiritual Guide and Visionary

We may not often think of this category as one fitting into the healing arts, but it definitely has that capacity. To be whole, we must be well in body, mind, and spirit. Thus, the spiritual guide and visionary serves the last part of the human trinity.

These people have an uncommon awareness of universal truths and how to communicate those lessons to a variety of people. Their statements are not dogmatic, but ring of authenticity and authority. They always remind us that spirituality is a central part of everyday living.

Many visionaries aspire to be part of this world, but not "of" it. In other words, they strive to teach us how to be true to our ideals while still coping with reality. They engender sparks in our dormant gifts, see through our facades, and inspire the best in us. Their gift is healing, nurturing, and motivating the struggling spirit through word and deed.

The position of guide and visionary is not always as wonderful as it sounds. Like Jesus in Gethsemane, visionaries sometimes feel forsaken by their students, the world, and even the gods themselves. Their responsibilities are heavy, and thus the lessons they learn personally are equally difficult and profound. They must somehow translate this learning into their teachings, while striving to continue their own spiritual growth.

Perhaps this is why the guide/visionary has historically led a hermetic existence. Here, people must seek them out. Here, they aren't pressured to provide wise insights all the time. Until found, they can remain alone with their thoughts and the divine.

The temptation to withdraw from the very people you hope to serve is the major drawback for the guide. To avoid this, try periodic retreats instead—times when you refill the well of self. Promise yourself a vacation, somewhere where people don't know you, and really rest. Rediscover the voice of the Sacred Parent during the silent moments, and let that energy carry you back to the world ready to serve once more.

Type 6: Gaia's Servants

The Earth needs healing, too. The ravages of greed and ignorance have left her scarred and weary. The soil in many regions is barren, animals are dying, and the water and air are polluted. Without wholeness in Gaia, people can never be whole. It is for this reason that I've included this unique healing art in this book.

The task of Gaia's servants is to keep the body of Earth healthy while rejuvenating its ailing spirit. People born to this group tend to have natural green thumbs, a kinship with animals, and an attunement to weather patterns and seasonal cycles. They use this awareness to work with the planet on a physical level.

Farmers were probably the Earth's first servants. They tend the soil with loving hands, giving back to the planet as much as possible of what they are given. Now, for the most part, that job is left to ecologically-minded folk.

Gaia's servants today are, in many ways, part pagan and part naturalist in their love for the living world. They recognize that humanity may become an endangered species if our approach toward the planet doesn't change. They also remind us that we have to learn how to play more safely and peacefully together in the sandbox called Earth. These are the people you see tenaciously recycling, setting up compost heaps, using natural bug repellents, picking up litter in the parks, helping endangered species, picketing against chemical dumping, supporting international cooperation, and hugging trees.

Gaia's servants give their greatest public exhibitions on Earth Day. Unfortunately, one day a year is not enough exposure to keep communities motivated the other 364. Therefore, ecological groups have begun political campaigns, year-round recycling collections, and other local/international efforts to clean up the human act. It is a tough job in which they have to fight the system and red tape every step of the way.

Earth-healers reach out toward the spirit of Gaia. Through meditation, visualization, and other New Age techniques, they hope to rekindle the vital spark in our planetary soul—quite literally loving the world into wellness. This particular task is one with which anyone (healer or not) can help.

Plant a seed and watch it grow. As you tend that greenery, name your seed "Earth" and extend the energy of joy, peace, and love toward the growing seedling. Drop a couple of blessed crystals in the soil, or use a natural fertilizer. All the while, allow the gentle nature of your care to move out from that plant like a wave to wrap the Earth in warmth.

In the process, a personal reciprocity with nature is brought back into your life, and you are also indirectly helping people. I remember a song I once heard early in my metaphysical studies. I believe it has Native American roots. It says: "It's sacred ground we walk upon, with every step we take." In effect, Gaia's servants are creating this hallowed ground upon which all people can flourish in the future.

Et Cetera

Healers of all walks and paths are part of the vision of a better tomorrow. Through our applied studies, we are helping develop a world where dis-ease is replaced by creative minds, vital bodies, and fulfilled spirits.

In the end, healing is not about power, money, fame, or glory. It is about helping. It is encompassed in those magical moments when we reach beyond ourselves to say, "I care. How can I help?" It is the lonely hand held through the night, a hot herbal tea to ease the discomforts of a friend, and sometimes even the smiles given to strangers. Once you become a practicing healer, people may never remember your face or name, but they will *always* remember the keepsake you leave behind: wholeness. What a tremendous gift to give each other and our world.

SELF-HELP REVIEW FOR CHAPTER 1

Did you answer several of the questions in the beginning of this chapter affirmatively, or perhaps see yourself in any of the personal accounts given by healers in this section? If so, were you able to discern for what areas of healing you might be most suited (types 1 through 6)? Keep this information in mind as you read the remainder of the book. It will help you find the right outlet for your talents.

If you did not answer yes, or feel any harmonic affinity with the healing types discussed in this chapter, that doesn't mean you cannot learn to heal. It just means you have no currently available foundation on which to build your abilities. In this instance, the remainder of this book furnishes the beginnings of that foundation and provides sound information so that you can choose a path and focus wisely.

In either case, don't give up on yourself or your desire to learn. Nothing that is worth doing, or that is truly lasting, is instantaneous. Patience, tenacity, determination, and compassion are the keys to achieving your goal of hands-on healing.

Healing: Accountability and Ethics

Over the library door in Thebes
is the inscription, "Medicine for the soul."
—Diodorus Siculus

TO UNDERSTAND THE TRADITIONAL ROLE OF healers and how that role affects modern practices, we must roll back the pages of time. In ancient civilizations, healers shouldered the burdensome task of being health educators while overcoming the prevalent superstitions of the time. During the early Middle Ages, when commoners considered baths unhealthy, for example, healers had to find ways to breach that barrier.

In matters like this, healers acted as both priest and physician, gently guiding their patients toward what they hoped was the best available cure. Historically speaking, medicine and religion walked hand in hand up until 100 years ago, because the origins of many sicknesses remained illusive. Indeed, except for the efforts of Hippocrates, who tried to take healing out of the hands of the gods and put it into those of the healer, the superstitious populace regarded matters of life and death as being mostly attributable to the whims of greater powers.

Except for monks, who studied and documented herbalism, which itself had "divine" origins, the Church was more than happy to foster such notions if they aided conversions and tithes. Even within the monastery, traditional mystical formulas mixed liberally with the new god on the scene, with the only change in many folk remedies being the replacement of a pagan god or goddess' name with that of Jesus, an archangel or the Virgin Mary. Thus, healers had to poise themselves carefully between what was deemed medically or socially correct, religiously proper, and emotionally sound in order to be truly effective in this setting.

Metaphysical healers also served individuals who shunned "new fangled" medicines, those seeking "miracles," or those hoping to experience something supernatural. This often made the healer's implied responsibility very weighty. This role and responsibility is no less great today.

While we have acquired a tremendous amount of medical knowledge, we have far more laws and regulations by which to abide. The overall public awareness of and concern about alternative medicine makes for a skeptical audience, yet this same audience is hungry for true spirituality, as evidenced by the popularity of New Age ideals. There also exists an undercurrent of discontent toward the medical profession for its sometimes seemingly inhumane treatment of patients—patients who then turn their hopes toward alternative methods.

No matter the reason, alternative healers are really battling the same dis-eases as those of old. Their quest is still making people whole. Now all that remains is accepting, empowering, and acting on that conviction in a responsible manner.

ACCEPTING YOUR HEALING GIFTS

It is not easy to accept and integrate spiritual abilities. To be truly effective in the healing arts however, this is the first step that must occur. It reminds me of the childhood game where you close your eyes and fall backward into a companion's hands. This requires tremendous trust and faith in that individual's ability to catch you and keep you safe from harm. With healing, there are no waiting hands or companions. The only person to trust is yourself.

So, the process of studying, accepting, and empowering healing abilities is often slow and steady. Like a child learning to walk, you must find your balancing point, having caution in one hand and confidence in the other. This is one of the reasons I suggest that my students begin practicing with close friends or family members at first. They will always give you honest feedback, and not judge harshly the minor errors that come from inexperience.

For example, healers using massage therapy may find their touch is too hard or too soft for their patient, and then over-compensate. They also might rush through the session, never really giving the individual time to adjust to the energies involved. Neither mistake completely negates the benefit of the effort, but these types of errors do get corrected with patience and practice.

Either way, the first step in healing is embracing your desire to heal with a welcoming heart. As scary as this step may seem, it is also a very rewarding one. You have found something sacred within yourself—an ability that reaches beyond your singleness to touch others. Rejoice in this new awareness.

Once you pass this juncture, life will change in unexpected and amazing ways. Healing energy does not only affect those whom you aid. It flows through and transforms you. Thus, your life, thoughts, and awareness all slowly adjust to reflect that marvelous growth.

THE HEALER'S TALISMAN

Once you reach this juncture, consider finding a token that represents your art. You can energize and bless this token like an amulet to aid your healing efforts, then carry or wear it regularly. In ancient times, a talisman was defined as images of a figure, character, or constellation placed on sympathetic stones or metals, often containing astrological correspondences. This was always executed purposefully to "affix" magic with the image.

You can simply expand this definition to include practical and easily obtainable items that are emblematic or useful in your methodology. Since you choose and bless this token, *you* become the single-minded "workman" de Brésche mentioned. Beyond the finished product, however, there are numerous benefits to the fashioning process.

First, the thought required in selecting an emblem helps us reassess our deepest feelings about becoming healers and the specific technique we have chosen. Like the flash of creative insight experienced and expressed by artists, the essence of your craft is about to be distilled into one medium (the token). In metaphysical beliefs, emblems are no less powerful than what they represent, so this should be a well-considered choice.

Symbols are also important to mental states when enacting any healing energies, because they activate our super-conscious instincts. Here the symbol tells our higher selves that something important is about to occur. This notification then serves to prepare our minds so they shift smoothly to an appropriate awareness level for the work ahead.

Using auric healing as an example, my talisman is an antique box with an air-tight lid that stores anointing oil. I only use this oil for auric balancing. When I take the container from its spot on the bookshelf, my mind immediately recognizes the intended application. The minute I grasp that box, I have essentially given nonverbal permission for my hands to go "on-line" as universal conduits once more.

I am also, by my actions, accepting the role of healer for the duration of this effort. Many healers find that it is not always easy to separate themselves from their art. Yet, in order to fulfill other mundane responsibilities, sometimes the mantle must be laid aside. In the few seconds it takes to lift my oil jar, I symbolically take up that mantle again in all its force.

In this illustration, the scent of the oils also provides a spiritual cue that effectively prepares and sets my whole atti- tude. This conditioned reaction didn't happen over night. It took several months of consistently using the same "rit- ual," but now it's very natural.

Another function of talismans is to help in maintaining concentration. For example, it seems that animals, espe- cially cats, love auric work. They gather around the healer and patient like an enraptured audience. Sometimes cats will walk over the patient to get closer to the action. In- stances like this become very distracting. Here, looking at (or holding) your chosen symbol while taking a deep, cleansing breath focuses your attention back on relevant matters.

Here is a brief list of some healing tokens I've seen. You may choose from this list, or find something else to try that is personally meaningful:

Crystals on chains for mediums, readers, auric bal- ancers, and crystal healers;

Ring or other "bobble" with inscribed runes for divin- ers, crystal healers, meditation;

Specific musical accompaniment used according to its theme for guided meditations, visualizations, and many other types of healing;

Special clothing or hair style used *only* during a heal- ing: color therapists, spells, and rituals;

A symbolically colored or scented basket of greenery for herbalists, holisticians, aroma therapists, color therapists;

A unique candle holder for past-life regressions (candles make excellent focals for this), meditation, and rebirthing;

An easily transported personal "charm," like a lucky penny, that you hold while concentrating;

Special artwork placed in the direct line of sight of the healer;

Incenses, oils, colognes, or perfumes chosen for their symbolic meaning;

Dowsing rods to discern the trouble areas for diviners and auric balancers.

One final note: it is not essential that you find a talisman to use as part of your healer's kit. Tools are just that: items that help us accomplish tasks more effectively. If you are uncomfortable with the idea, or can't seem to find the right symbol, trust your instincts. As with all matters of spirituality, let the inner voice be your ultimate guide and decision maker.

AN ACCEPTANCE RITUAL

People have always marked distinctive occurrences with special observances. On our day of birth, we hold a party that acknowledges the spirit of life. When children are born, we set aside a name day to welcome them and thank the divine for such a wonderful gift. Accepting your graduation into practicing the healing arts is equally worthy of commemoration.

The information that follows is an example only. Exactly what you do to acknowledge your new role is purely a personal decision. I have included this here as an outline for those who want to have a distinctive observance, but are uncertain as to where to begin their planning. Please add your vision and creativity to this in heaping quantities for the most pleasing and meaningful results.

I urge caution and careful consideration before entering into such a ritual, however. The commitment you're about to accept is a serious one. It is a pledge that you make to the god/dess, to others, and to yourself (see "Discovering Healing Talents," p. 8). Such promises are not entered into lightly or without knowledge of the duties that will follow. Don't dive into this pool before looking closely at its contents. Take your time and think about what this moment means to you. Seek out other healers for their advice. Wait until you feel 100 percent certain that this path is right for you, then move forward with a joyful heart.

The Ritual

Timing: During a full Moon for maturity and abundant energy.

Setting: The area where you wish to do most of your healing work. Alternatively, any location with deep personal significance relative to this moment.

Accoutrements: If you're going to use special clothing or jewelry regularly in your art, wear it now, or have it ready to don as part of the ritual.

Decorations: Any appropriate symbols or "tools of the trade." Green candles for rejuvenation, energizing pieces of art, live plants to symbolize growth, other personal items that engender thoughts of transition and change. If you have a specific divine visage that you honor regularly, keep an emblem of it nearby.

Incense: Consider traditionally healthful or cleansing scents like pine, lavender (for rest), allspice, rosemary, bay, and lilac (for energy). Another option is nutmeg to increase spiritual awareness. To make these burn evenly on self-lighting charcoal, blend ¼ cup of powdered wood with ½ tsp. of each herb desired.

Sprinkle lightly over the heated coals in a fire-proof container.

Attendees: Not necessary. If you have been trained by someone, they will probably want to participate. You can also invite special friends or family members who can empower you with their love and support. In this case, they should stand around you in a circle, visualizing the green light of healing filling the room.

Prayer: Sometimes it is best to write these ahead of time, or just speak openly from your heart. However, for those who would like an example to modify for personal use, I include the following:

Spirit of love, light, and life, I come before you today in the role of a servant; one who receives the knowledge and gifts you have given with a grateful heart. Help me to begin learning my craft today, so that I can ease the suffering of _____ (animals, people, the Earth). Allow my hands to be always gentle and welcoming, my heart sensitive and caring, and my eyes open to see needs wherever they may be. Guide my hands in the healing arts from this day forward. So let it be.

This type of prayer is a nice way to end the ritual, as it provides closure.

Activities: Again, this is a personal choice depending on what seems most meaningful and appropriate to you. I offer these as ideas for your consideration:

1. Bless and consecrate the token spoken of earlier in this chapter. Use words and movements customary to your path, and with which you are comfortable.

2. Make a special outfit that you can put on during your ritual to symbolically don your new role in the healing arts.

3. Have any friends or family members express their feelings at this moment, including their hopes for you personally.

4. Offer to use your gifts for the benefit of those attending, so you can start practicing.

5. Have the room sectioned off into two separate halves, so you can move from one to the other as an emblem of transformation. Alternatively, step over a line, broom handle, or candle to mark the transition.

6. Burn, bury, or otherwise ritually destroy an emblem of the "old" self. This effectively tells the universe that you are willing to leave outworn ideas and ways behind you. This is also an excellent time to rid yourself of any nonhealthy personal habits, like smoking. Remember that part of a healer's job is being a role model.

7. Have a specially prepared meal afterward, consisting of healthy, revitalizing items like raw vegetable platters and breads with honey. If possible, choose foods for their metaphoric value, like making a vanilla yogurt dip with almond and serving apple juice, both of which symbolize well-being.

8. Post-ritual reveling! This is a time to celebrate and remember. Take a moment for some good kinship, conversation, and relaxation.

EMPOWERING YOUR TALENTS

You have bravely and boldly stepped into your new role as a healer. Now what? Even among the most schooled of these arts, there are no comprehensive manuals to follow and no rules carved in stone. This can be rather disconcerting, to say the least.

First, know that experience is a terrific teacher, one that is only harsh when you don't pay attention. The more often you use your knowledge and skills, the better developed both become. Your sensitivity to metaphysical energy increases each time you work with an open mind and heart.

As you walk this new pathway, keep a diary of your experiences to help gauge your growth. If you read this every couple of months, I can nearly promise you will see positive signs of increasing maturity and talent mingled with your words. This in itself is empowering, but may not be enough, depending on the depth of need you face daily. That is when energizing activities become beneficial and sometimes essential to success.

ENERGIZING ACTIVITIES

These sample exercises prepare and revitalize individuals for their healing art(s). The idea is to bring the mind, body, and spirit into symmetry so sacred energy can flow more smoothly. Exactly how each person achieves this peaceful state can vary greatly depending on personality, the type of healing, or the environment. Please change, combine, or adapt these activities so they better suit your needs and circumstances.

Meditation and Visualization

This very popular method only requires a place to sit and the ability to concentrate with single-mindedness. Close your eyes and take a deep cleansing breath in through your nose, breathing out through your mouth. Let the burdens of the day fall from your shoulders to be absorbed by the Earth. Release your tensions, your worries, and enjoy the quiet, reassuring sound of your heartbeat.

Next, begin to visualize the air around you as filled with brilliant, sparkling light. Breathe this air into each cell and membrane of your being, then exhale all the negativity it collects there. You will probably see this as thick, brownish light when you exhale. Continue in this manner until the light exhaled is as clean as that inhaled. This means you've released your negativity and are ready to work.

Finally, fill yourself with the light of healing. Most people say it's easiest to visualize this coming down from the heavens, first into your head, then into your heart, and finally out through your hands (or tool of your art). The color of the light should equate to health in your mind, vibrant green being most popular. Let this saturate your entire body until you feel ready to burst. If desired, you may continue this visualization as part of your healing technique.

Centering Exercise

For people who have trouble with visualization, this centering exercise, combined with meditation, often helps. You will need a chime, a bell, or a Tibetan prayer bowl for this activity.

Begin by getting comfortable somewhere where you can have the chime, bell, or bowl within reach. Begin in the same manner as the meditation above, but instead of visualizing light, sound the bowl/bell with each breath you take. Feel the vibrations of that sound as they surround and fill you with energy. Allow every portion of your being to resonate with that wave of power.

Some people who use this method routinely taperecord slow steady chime strokes instead, so they can focus all their attention on the sound. With this, consider adding brief affirmative phrases like, "I am holy," or, "I am a waiting vessel." Sometimes healers play this tape while working.

In this case, they direct the sound waves through their tool(s) and toward the patient, instead of accepting it into themselves.

Sacred Sounds[1]

The sacred word of creation brought all things into existence. In John 1:1, the biblical writer implies that this word and the divine force are one and the same power. It is this word power that sacred sounds try to capture and utilize.

In Hinduism, the "AUM" chant is a perfect example. This tone equates to the threefold divine name. By repeating it, chanters bring themselves into perfect harmony with that essence, within and without.

In the *Encyclopedia of Ancient and Forbidden Knowledge*, Zolar said: "The ability to make and change the mind dwells within."[2] This means that, through our use of sacred sounds or personally meaningful phrases, we can transform our mindset in preparation for healing. By repeating brief sounds or phrases, we accept the energy of change that they represent, then manifest this by opening our hearts and spirits to higher powers. Once this symmetry is achieved, divine energy flows more freely and naturally.

If you would like to study more on this topic, I suggest reading *Words of Power*, by Brain and Ester Crowley. In the meantime, the Hindu "AUM" or the phrase "I am" both work very well. The former encourages unity with your own higher self or the sacred powers, while the latter reaffirms your importance in the universe.

Most often, chanting, mantras, and toning are done in combination with meditation. Through this blending, the

---

[1]See also "Sound Therapy," chapter 17.
[2]Zolar, *Encyclopedia of Ancient and Hidden Knowledge* (New York: Fireside/ Simon & Schuster, 1989).

sound waves accentuate deeper states of awareness and promote a ready, open vessel.

Sacred Movement

Throughout the ancient and modern world, we have solid examples of the use of sacred movement for religious or spiritual purposes. The whirling dervish dancers of a Muslim ascetic order use circular dances as part of divinatory attempts. Sufi dancers employ specific, rhythmic movements to increase their awareness of natural orders and cycles and bring healing to the planet. In the Old Testament, priests and worshippers danced before the Ark of the Covenant as a form of worship.

In *Sacred Dance,* W. O. E. Oesterly shows that movement was essential to many early rituals. For many ancient civilizations, dancing was a way to achieve unity with the divine. Oesterly writes: "By associating yourself with it, you are already in an indefinable way, in communion with it."[3] Thus, movement is an alternative vehicle for obtaining and depicting oneness with the Great Spirit.

Sacred movement is not limited to the realms of dance and the preparation process. I have many friends who interpret for the deaf. In watching them, I realize that the beauty of each hand movement and the visual form created is truly marvelous. Add to this natural talent a little positive energy, and a gift for hypnotism could conceivably develop. This talent could then be applied in healing to help overcome habits and negative thought forms.

Another example is massage. In observing a masseuse who has achieved an altered state of awareness, you see that their gestures evidence a unique sensitivity to the patient. Each stroke appears to flow naturally into the next, thereby

---

[3]W. O. E. Oesterly, *Sacred Dance* (Cambridge, MA: Cambridge University Press, 1923).

aiding overall effectiveness. In this manner, therapists allow their unity with universal powers to express itself through movement. Here, and in the previous illustration, movement is a medium for healing energy that also aids the healer's concentration, thereby allowing energy to flow without interference.

The Ritual Bath

Water is a potent symbol in many traditions. Christians baptize their children at birth to cleanse them, bring wholeness, and invoke divine blessings. Wiccans sprinkle water around a magic circle's participants to deter negative energy. In Britain, there are hundreds of sacred wells believed to have indwelling water spirits that will aid supplicants.

The ritual bath is an offshoot of these ideas. It embraces water's cleansing symbolism as a means to prepare for healing. Here, healers discard mundane clothing and rinse away any negative feelings or tensions that could potentially disrupt their work. Next, they allow the lunar nature of water to "tickle" their own auric energy into an aware state. The ritual has an additional benefit in that it can be executed *after* a session to wash away any lingering energy remnants.

A ritual bath may be taken by patients to relieve excess negativity, improve relaxation, and generally prepare them for the work ahead (see chapter 9).

Cyclical Breathing

Nearly every class taught on meditation includes examples of good breathing techniques to improve the ability to concentrate. By focusing on our vital breath, we begin to retrain our minds to think about only one thing instead of hundreds. These exercises also improve our awareness of self in body and spirit.

Cyclical breathing connects each breath to the next, creating a circle of air within and around you. In effect, it can become a mystical sphere of energy for cleansing, protection, or rejuvenation. To accomplish this, take a deep breath (in through your nose) and begin filling the region around your navel with air until you feel comfortably full. Then slowly release this breath from your mouth, in a gentle constant stream. Just as you run out of air, begin the next cycle.

To this technique, add the light visualization mentioned earlier or other meditative methods that you find helpful. This is an especially good exercise if you're having trouble sleeping. In this case, lie in bed focusing all your attention on slow, rhythmic breaths. Allow any tensions picked up from healing (or worries of the day) to be blown away when you exhale. Then, take in the fresh winds of change! You will awaken very refreshed and ready to begin anew.

COUNTERING ENERGY DRAINS

The above exercises improve our ability to heal without too much personal depletion. However, tremendous amounts of energy can be channeled during healings, at least some of which may be personal. To offset unnecessary exhaustion, consider the following:

1. Take regular "down time" from healing for relaxing diversions. Go for a long walk and allow nature to absorb your weariness. Swim or perform other physical actions to relieve stress. Read a good book that has nothing to do with healing, or even take a nap.

2. Remember that you are a conduit for power. While some personal involvement is necessary, you don't

have to expend only personal energy on your gifts. Let the divine/universal stream move through you freely. Don't try to do it alone. The more you "let go and let god," the less tiring healing becomes.

3. You have the right, and sometimes the responsibility, to say "no." None of us can be all things to all people. If you don't feel up to the work, it's best to decline gracefully. This shows a respect for your own well-being and that of your patient.

4. Make metaphysically invigorating or educational activities part of your daily routine. Just like the body, our spirits need regular exercise to function well.

5. Network with other healers in your field, and find a few to whom you can send your patients when you are unable to work (see also #3 above). This way, you can really relax without feeling guilty about those whose needs you could not meet effectively.

HEALING AS A SERVICE

Ultimately, when you accept your role as a healer, you become a leader among a close-knit group of people. People will naturally be drawn to your side because of the comforting energies you exude. Consequently, folks will sometimes come to you for aid in matters having nothing whatsoever to do with health.

Sometimes this means stepping out of your traditional healing niche into other areas. If you are an auric healer, you may find some proficiency at reading past lives, for example, but you must recognize your limitations. There is nothing wrong with telling people that their request is not within the range of your abilities. In fact, this is responsible service.

Also, remember that service can be abused. Your gifts should not be "volunteered" by others or used as entertainment. People naturally desire spiritual experiences, but sometimes they don't realize how taxing they can be. In their exuberance, they may tell friends about your talents and offer a demonstration without consulting you. Suddenly you find yourself in an awkward spot.

When moments like this arise, first consider the circumstances. If it is obvious that these people are just looking for a diversion, you can always politely decline. There is nothing that says a healer's compassion has to equate to lenience. You have every right to decide when and where your art is exercised.

On the other hand, there may be a real need to address. If so, and you feel prepared to help, proceed. Later, take your good-intentioned friend aside and point out that it's not "cool" to presume such services without at least asking first. Usually this avoids the problem in the future.

Use these occasions as an opportunity to educate the group gathered. Let them know you don't normally enact such procedures in public because of the sacredness of your work. Then explain what you're doing, so they begin to understand the nature of alternative medicine.

Finally, service is something that sees a need and responds to it. When you walk this path, you become an example. This means picking up litter, helping an elderly person with grocery bags, and enacting other small, meaningful gestures whose only rewards are the thanks of the recipients. These actions seem, superficially, to have nothing to do with healing. Yet, in spirit, they have everything to do with metaphysical ideals.

Without a caring attitude, it is difficult for healing gifts to function at their best, if at all. Our lives will often speak louder than our words. When people see us consistently acting in a manner befitting our spiritual path, they respond by respecting and trusting us more. This builds a positive atmosphere in which healers can serve the community more effectively.

There is also an additional bonus to our efforts. By making our lives an act of worship, we consistently renew our pledge to the Sacred Parent to make this world a better place. We also reiterate that commitment to our own hearts.

The Healers' Code

New Age healers quest for wholeness. Yet this is not a savage, "rules be damned" mission. To be true to spiritual ideals, healers must adhere to certain codes that protect both the healer and the patient.

While each person must determine his or her own guidelines, please read this section with an open mind and heart. From my own work, and those of people I deeply respect, the following list has been assembled. I think you will find it helpful and thought-provoking.

1. Ours is to heal, not to harm. This means doing everything in your power to help the natural healing process without endangering the individual. For example, a wise herbalist or holistician never tells patients to forego their physician's orders. Instead, these gifts are added in sensitive harmony with modern science for the greatest benefit.

2. Except in emergency situations, you should always obtain permission for healing. Never intrude on another's free will. When emergencies arise, seek divine counsel and consult your own inner voice for guidance. Consider the spiritual dimension here—the karmic reprise—should any such knowledge or abilities get used for the wrong reasons.

3. If one can cure, two can kill; be careful with your gifts and use them wisely. We live in a world where more equates to better. This is rarely the case with hands-on healing. Instead, quality is far preferred to quantity.

4. Gentleness and kindness are valuable commodities. Remember to treat the problem with ferocity, but treat the patient as a person. The patient is not the disease.

5. Remember, you're human too. You can not give wholly of yourself when you're sick, angry, or otherwise out of sorts.

6. Never work when you can not put aside negative personal feelings toward the individual in need. In holistic treatments, anger can translate into making a malady worse instead of better.

7. You are a counselor and friend, too. Sometimes the greatest gift a healer can provide is a good ear and a little personalized attention.

8. **This is important.** Legally speaking, you are not a doctor, nor may you make any claims of medical qualities to your efforts, other than those afforded by licensing. This is especially true of herbalists whose preparations are consumed by their clients. Generally, it is best to label your services "for amusement only," and explain the limitations to your clients in detail. This will keep you from inadvertently committing fraud—a federal offense.

9. You must love something to make it whole. This means loving your art and extending that joy with your knowledge and abilities.

10. **(Optional)** Read the Hippocratic Oath periodically. Hippocrates was one of the first visionaries to put the responsibility for medical treatment (and its outcome) into the hands of the healers themselves. He said: "I swear by Apollo Physician, by Asclepias, by Health, by Panacea and by all the gods and goddesses, making them my witness, that I will carry out, according to my ability and judgement, this oath and this indenture . . . I will keep pure and holy both my life and my art. In whatsoever houses I enter, I will enter to help the sick . . ." His words still hold tremendous wisdom today.

11. To be an effective healer, you can not only treat the symptoms, but must root out the cause of the problem, including those of mind and spirit. Otherwise, the condition will recur.

12. If you work with love and good intentions, you can always help others, with or without a tremendous amount of skill.

13. If patients do not truly want to be whole, no amount of effort on your part will change their fate. Everyone must be somewhat responsible for their own wellness. You are only a helpmate.

14. Keep thorough records of your work, including referrals. Network with other healers to get new, refreshing ideas. Speak with organizations who support your field and find out the legalities of practicing in your region.

15. Never lose sight of the fact that you are treating unique individuals with unique problems—don't start categorizing out of laziness.

16. Allow your vision to shine through your work. Healing offers each of us a unique opportunity to express our spiritual sensitivity while helping other human beings. No matter how dramatic the exterior results may be, the interior effects of such caring moments are not to be underestimated.

USING THIS BOOK

The remainder of this text is set up as an informational source, describing the history, techniques, and legalities of various New Age healing methods. Each section can help you with several things, including:

1. Explaining the background of various methods to people new to metaphysical healing;

2. Exploring additional or alternative healing methods to apply in your own work;

3. Examining (or experimenting with) other techniques, about which you may be interested or curious;

4. Building your own personal knowledge of New Age healing approaches so you can communicate these ideas to people seeking aid;

5. Examining other procedures to discern if you have a natural aptitude for that specific healing technique;

6. Examining procedures that you may wish to incorporate into your own regimen for personal well-being.

Beyond all this, there is the wonderful diversity and beauty of New Age healing to investigate. Each of the methods presented seeks to unify the divine nature with physical reality to improve the quality of life. And, in truth, isn't that what all positive spiritual paths should strive to do?

SELF-HELP REVIEW FOR CHAPTER 2

How do you view your role as a healer today versus the role of healers in history? Specifically, in what ways are your feelings similar to or different from what you think theirs may have been?

Were you able to find a talisman for your technique, or a symbol to use regularly? If so, what did you choose and why?

What activities of those given were best for energizing you, and for countering energy drains? Did you change or personalize these in any way to make them more effective?

Can you think of any more ethical guidelines to add to your personal healer's code? If so, what?

The hands that heal are also those that love. They are those inspiring us to recognize every moment of every day as special and a divine privilege. Hands-on healing also inspires a renewed awareness that our health is one of the greatest gifts we have. I pray these pages become part of that heritage.

Part II

Techniques

*A physician should be a servant of Nature,
and not her enemy; he should be able to
guide and direct her in her struggle for life and
not throw, by his unreasonable interference,
fresh obstacles in the way of recovery.*
—Paracelsus, *The Paragranum*

1

Acupressure and Acupuncture

> *We are proposing welcoming the body back
> into unison with the self.*
> —Rollo May

ACUPUNCTURE IS AT LEAST TWO THOUSAND YEARS old. Scrolls dating from 200 B.C. describe the foundational principles of acupuncture and the use of moxibustion (discussed later this section). From these records, we learn of a doctor in the 4th century B.C. named Bia Que who used acupuncture to heal a coma patient. Bia Que also provided the foundational system of diagnosis for acupuncture—that of watching, listening, smelling, inquiring, and touching.

As we study this ancient art, we must bear in mind that acupressure is also a philosophical system that sees people as multidimensional beings—having both body and spirit. Unlike Western medicine, which is linear (e.g. cause—cure), the goal of acupuncture and acupressure is to get all aspects of the human dimensions working together harmoniously, including those that go beyond the physical (holistic).

In treating diseases, Western medicine uses medication, whereas acupuncture and acupressure focus their energies on improving the body's ability to resist sickness.[1]

---

[1]Time-Life Books, eds. *Powers of Healing* (Alexandria, VA: Time-Life Books, 1989), p. 50.

Consequently, there are few ailments for which acupuncture and acupressure don't offer some type of defense. The World Health Organization lists forty illnesses that acupuncture is capable of treating, including bronchitis and diarrhea. Additionally, even Western medicine recognizes its beneficial effects as a nonnarcotic alternative to pain medication. Acupuncture and acupressure have both exhibited high levels of success in easing toothache, headache, and painful muscle or joint conditions without drugs.

Acupuncture and acupressure have roots deep in Chinese Taoism. In this tradition, the body represents the dynamic middle ground between heavenly and Earthly energies. For a person to be fully healthy, balance must be maintained between these two. Each organ in the body has a specific function in this symmetry, as do all our actions, thoughts, and habits. Anything that is contrary to the *Dao* (or way in which the Universe works) cannot abide—when people are not living in harmony with the *Dao,* dis-ease occurs.

Healers who study these arts are taught that the body is self-healing; that all people are capable of being regenerated from within. After all, our bodies perform hundreds of functions daily. We grow, we digest food, bruises heal—all without our intimate attention. Thus, the healer's job is not healing directly. Instead, the goal is to reconstruct positive universal energy patterns with which the patient's own healing capacity can work beneficially.

There are some immediate effects from both arts, but ultimately, the healer aims at marshalling physical and spiritual energies into long-term stability so their efforts will no longer be necessary. So much is this the case that Chinese custom dictates that the physician is paid only when the patient is *well;* payments cease with the onset of disease.

Acupressure and acupuncture are guided by the same basic principles. They both regard each part of the body as being *yin* (feminine) or *yang* (masculine), and as aligned to

Table 1. Acupressure and Acupuncture Associations.				
ELEMENT	THEME	SEASON	POLARITY	ORGAN
Wood	Renewal	Spring	Masculine	Liver
Fire	Transforming energy	Summer	Masculine to extreme	Heart
Earth	Growth; foundation	Early Fall	Balanced	Pancreas
Metal	Maturity; fulfillment	Autumn	Feminine	Lungs
Water	Repose; sleep	Winter	Feminine to extreme	Kidneys

one of the five elements that compose the universal matrix (fire, wood, earth, metal, water). Table 1 gives a brief overview of these associations.

Both also use specific points called *tsubos* which lie along a patient's physical meridians for guiding and opening any blocked pathways. Meridians are basically like Ley lines (see "Sacred Geometry," p. 161) on the Earth, only they connect the body's energy centers into a pattern. There are twelve primary meridians that end in the toes and fingers, each of which corresponds to a primary internal organ. Along the meridians, 365 acupuncture points exist, and it is likely no coincidence that this number corresponds to the total number of days in the year—a full cycle.

If a *tsubo* is blocked or shut down for some reason, it is the healer's job to recognize that problem and begin removing the obstruction. Illness occurs due to these blockages, which restrict the free flow of *chi*. In acupressure, fingers are applied to the *tsubo*, while in acupuncture, the healer uses a needle. The size of this needle, the depth which it penetrates, and whether or not it is manipulated after insertion depend upon the condition.

People in both acupuncture and acupressure will often test each *tsubo* for evidence of discomfort. Pain equates to blockage. So, when the finger or needle activates that center by its presence, it frees the *chi* and the pain should abate. While healers work, they will often recommend that a patient use deep breathing to ease discomfort and liberate the energy.

In any case, the healer attempts to reestablish an even flow of *chi*, which is required for health regulation. Here, the body is like a musical score that the healer adjusts and then plays, until it is "just right." In many ways, this adjustment is not so different from regular car tune-ups—except that the spiritual nature replaces the mechanical.

Something else that sometimes accompanies acupuncture is moxibustion. In this procedure, a lump of moxa (mugwort) on top of a piece of ginger gets added to one end of the acupuncture needle. After the healer inserts the needle, the moxa is ignited, which warms the needle and stimulates *chi*. Today, several alternatives to moxibustion have developed. They include using laser beams instead of needles, the addition of mild electrical stimulation, injecting homeopathic solutions into an acupoint, and ultrasound.

Moxibustion illustrates an important point about acupuncture and acupressure. These are but two facets of the very large crystal of Chinese medicine. Acupuncture does not work in a vacuum. In the East, it is often accompanied by herbs, dietary regimens, exercise, and massage.[2] Acupuncture is also accompanied with a specific approach to diagnosis called the "four examinations."

To determine not only the origins of a problem, but the best treatment, acupuncturists touch, ask numerous questions, listen closely to their client's responses, and smell the body. Of these methods, touch is considered the

---

[2]Sonia Lopez, *Acupuncture* (New York: Harmony Books, 1988), p.15.

most important, including checking the twelve pulse points (six per wrist). As early as 2600 B.C., Chinese medicine advocated this pulse examination as the greatest determinant for diagnosis. Touch in other regions of the body also sets off sympathetic reactions (like sensitivity or mild pain) that tell the healer much about a patient's mental and physical state. With all this information gathered, the acupuncturist then sets to work.

Acupuncture is safe and has few side effects. Some people believe that it stimulates the nervous system so that the body releases natural analgesics and endorphins, thereby controlling pain. In China, acupuncture is often used in place of any painkillers during surgery and childbirth. Acupuncture has also proven itself beneficial for treating animals. Nonetheless, acupuncture is a very refined art that should never be undertaken by someone who has not been properly trained.

Some of the less complex systems of acupressure, however, are ones with which almost anyone can work with a little practice. By learning the meridians and pressure points, one can apply mild pressure for five seconds, then release and repeat. Pressure-point stimulation is a kind of massage, but very brief. Because of this, the legalities of practicing on anyone other than yourself or friends vary from region to region. Most remedial massage therapists must be licensed, but that doesn't lessen the potential for acupressure as a type of self-healing, or an avenue for potential study.

To begin, go to the area of the body recommended in Table 2 (page 54). Explore with your fingertip until you find a distinctly sensitive spot in that region. With your fingertip pointing downward, rub in a counterclockwise direction to begin opening the flow of *chi*. Repeat only if necessary, stopping when the symptom stops. While the problem may return in the future, it will not be as severe. Re-stimulate the same point again, remaining calm and relaxed as you do, and the frequency of the problem should slowly fade.

Table 2. Accupressure Points and Applications.

PRESSURE POINT	APPLICATION
Wrist, slightly above bulge, top side.	Colds and related symptoms, headaches, wrist problems.
Wrist, top side, just below center point, toward elbow.	Tension, cough, depression, wrist problems.
Wrist, inner; three fingers up from wrist moving toward inner elbow.	Heartburn, sleeplessness, headache, nerves, upset stomach, arm.
Wrist, inner; along line of thumb.	Eye problems, sleep disorders, headaches, nausea.
Arm, elbow, bend away from body.	Heat rash, itchy skin, shoulder problems, elbows.
Ankle, behind, toward back of leg.	Lower back, cramps, strains, toothaches.
Leg, lower; about a hand's width above inner ankle, behind shin.	Constipation, hangover, nausea—all types.
Leg, lower; hand's length below knee on tibia.	Bladder and colon, weariness, nausea, itching, rash, digestion.
Hand, on thumb, between nail and joint.	Hand, head, sinuses, sore throat, laryngitis.
Hand, back; between thumb and first finger crease.	Acne, face, forearms, lips, neck, relaxation, mouth—especially gums.

There are certain precautions to take, however. People who have chronic problems, who are on medication or highly agitated, or pregnant women past the first trimester should not work with this system, called G-Jo. Similarly, a point located on an injury or particularly sensitive body part should also be avoided.

There are other healing techniques that have some type of acupressure as their foundation. Shiatsu, for example, combines traditional acupressure with massage and touch therapy to improve circulation. Shiatsu translates as "finger pressure." It originated in Japan in the early 1900s, combining an ancient form of massage with Western manipulations.

The most important area for diagnosis in Shiatsu is the *hara*, or abdomen, where the individual's vital force abides. The Japanese believe the source of *ki* (same as Chinese *chi*) is the *hara*. Beyond this, there is a tremendous focus on breath in Shiatsu to connect the practitioner and patient and improve centering. Let's listen to a friend who practices a type of pressure-point therapy very similar to Shiatsu, but slightly more gentle.

Todd's Insights[3]

Pressure-point and deep massage is actually a tremendous gift for both the patient and healer. In essence, this approach allows you to connect with the Greater Self, the Collective Unconscious and the healer within. From this altered state of awareness, everything becomes intuitive—a deep knowingness that profoundly affects both people during the process.

The foundational belief system in this type of bodywork is that the muscles and nerves of our bodies remember everything we've experienced; everything we internalize. As a healer works with the pressure points, the objective is freeing those memories, and thereby opening the natural connective system to healthful energy. Blockage

---

[3]Used by permission. Todd Alan runs a wonderful jewelry business, with all custom-designed pieces, and other beautiful art. Write: Creations Gallery, 1685 Main St., Peninsula, OH 44264; 216-468-2097.

causes imbalance. Once the resistance is removed, wellness begins to be reestablished.

I find that my hands may itch or burn when someone nearby has a need, but I do not consider myself a professional healer. For me, this is a joyous gift that finds expression when Spirit decrees. It is also an interesting aside to note that the same Eastern techniques that allow for healing are also foundational to the martial arts— an interesting two-sided coin. Thus, one must be very careful in treating people, as harm can come if your attention wanders.

I can't stress enough how important it is to be in the "right space" for this type of healing. When you serve others, that service can be a difficult taskmaster to which you can give too much of yourself. By finding the right frame of mind, the energy is free to flow and you're less apt to drain personal reserves. Also, many people find that an exceedingly focused frame of mind is essential for helping their life partners. Here, objectivity gets muddled with emotion and concern.

Once healers begin working with pressure points, they may find patients need some reassurance to allow themselves to open up . . . to really feel. Past this point many things may occur. Be prepared for everything from laugher to tears and body tremors. This is just each person's body reacting differently to release. Comfort patients about this experience; encourage them to breath into it and through it . . . allow it to be. This is the first step on that person's path back to balance of body, mind, and spirit.

Polarity therapy, developed by Dr. Randolph Stone in the early 1900s, divides the body into positive and negative poles, the latter corresponding to the lower extremities and the left side (similar to meridians). The therapist then uses energy transmitted through the auric envelope to excite or sedate the poles, depending on the need. The healer accomplishes this relay by light touches to various areas of the body along with minor manipulations. The goal is to realign the body's posture and thereby maximize the patient's ability to heal.

Another related art, Jin Shin Do, also called Body Mind Acupressure, descends from techniques developed in the Buddhist temples of Tibet and China. A Japanese philosopher, Jiro Murai, rediscovered these techniques in the early 1900s, calling the art Jin Shin Jitsu. It was not practiced in the United States until the 1950s, and the Jin Shin Do Foundation was established in 1982 by Iona Marsaa Teeguarden. Ms. Teeguarden studied in Japan and the United States, and devised a system that is characterized by the use of firm direct pressure (address at the end of this section).

Jin Shin Do retains the original form of direct pressure, and unlike Jin Shin Jitsu, it combines classic acupressure QiGong (Chi Kung), and Reichian theory. The beginning student uses eight balancing meridians and fifty-five pressure points, out of hundreds used by a master, with the goal of opening the body's electromagnetic rivers so they flow unhindered. Each session lasts one to one-and-a-half hours.

Jin Shin Do is considered effective for stress relief because of the emotional release that comes from relaxing the body's armor. This armor builds over the years with internalization and tension. The practitioner works toward releasing that build-up, to increase the client's awareness of the body-mind connection. In some instances, this approach has proved so effective that the *East-West Journal* reported in August of 1985 that it successfully helped handicapped children over many hurdles in their rehabilitation.

The following addresses may prove useful if you want to explore various forms of acupunture or acupressure.

Jin Shin Do Foundation
1084 G. San Miguel
  Canyon Rd.
Watsonville, CA 95076-9135
Phone: 408-763-7702

Colorado School of Chinese
  Medicine (acupuncture)
1441 York St. #202
Denver, CO 80206-2127
Phone: 303-329-6355

APTA (Polarity Therapy)
2888 Bluff St., #149
Boulder, CO 80301
Phone: 303-545-2080

Shiatsu School of Canada
547 College St.
Toronto, Ontario M6G 1A9
Canada
Phone: 1-800-263-1703

Accupressure Institute
1533 Shattuck Ave.
Berkeley, CA 94709
Phone: 1-800-442-2232

Body Therapy Institute
Santa Barbara, CA
Phone: 805-966-5802

Body Therapy Center
368 California Ave.
Palo Alto, CA 94306
Phone: 415-328-9400

Tse Qigong Center
Manchester, England
Phone: 011 44 0161-929-
   4485
E-Mail: qimag@michaeltse.
   u-net.com

2

Aromatherapy

His orient beams, on herb, tree, fruit, and flower,
glistering with dew; fragrant the fertile Earth,
After soft showers; and sweet the coming on
Of grateful evening mild, then silent night. . . .
—John Milton

AROMATHERAPY IS VERY HOLISTIC AND HOMEO-
pathic in nature because of its subtlety. Scents affect us
every day, frequently without us ever being totally aware of
their effect. If you don't think this is true, just consider the
different emotions engendered by the smell of fresh-baked
bread and the morning pot of coffee versus gas fumes and
overheated garbage!

The ancients knew this distinctive human reaction
when they recommended leaving certain types of flowers,
like lavender, near the bedside of a sick person. The scent
abated sadness and therefore helped the patient's recuperation. In fact, chronicles dating back to the 1500 B.C. docu-
ment the use of aromatics like lavender in medicine.

The Egyptians used them for embalming their
pharaohs and for treating depression. Aromatics also
played a key role in religion, filling the temples of gods and
goddesses around the world. The Greeks even considered
aromatic herbs to be of divine origin. Babylonians put perfume in the blocks which were assembled into temples. In
India, this idea was further refined simply by making the
walls of the sacred space out of sandalwood panels.

Hippocrates recommended a daily aromatic bath for health. In the Middle Ages, healers burned resins to avert the plague. During the Victorian era, physicians often filled the top of their walking stick with pungent herbs for much the same reason. Interestingly enough, studies indicate that people who worked in perfume factories during epidemics had a higher survival rate than commonly expected! Today, many aromatics remain as a foundation to drugs prescribed in modern pharmaceuticals.

The term "aromatherapy" was coined about fifty years ago by a French chemist named Maurice Gottefosse. In truth, the French obsession with fine perfumes, dating back to the 12th century, is probably responsible for much of the initial progress in this field. Consider: Gottefosse published a book on this topic in France in 1928, while a fellow countryman named Jean Valnet started using aromatic cures as part of his treatments. Yet another biochemist from France, Marguerite Maury, used essential oils for massage, believing that, as they got absorbed into the skin, internal problems would also be treated![1] This created a solid foundation upon which our current aromatherapies continue to build.

Aromatherapists use essential oils that are distilled, expressed, or dissolved[2] in a medium from various flowers, fruits, leaves, seeds, roots, and trees. During the treatment process, these oils may be administered orally, through inhalation, or applied externally, external applications being

---

[1]Robert Tisserand, *The Art of Aromatherapy* (Rochester, VT: Healing Arts Press, 1977), p. 43.

[2]Distillation is done in large vats where a plant is steamed at high temperature. The vapor is then cooled which causes condensation, and the resulting oil is collected. Expression is basically squeezing or pressing as one does to a lemon rind to get juice. Finally, solvents like alcohol may be used for flowers where the high heat of distillation would evaporate the delicate oils. Later, the waxy oils are separated from the base to obtain what is called an "absolute." Absolute rose is still one of the most expensive perfumes known.

the most common and noninvasive. Because of its simple methods, aromatherapy is a perfect mate to modern, hectic schedules.

Aromatherapists return our attention to nature's medicine cabinet. Each oil has a physical, emotional, or spiritual effect, while some affect several levels of the human condition without chemicals. This means aromatics are Earth-friendly and people-friendly. Sage oil, for example, cleanses both physically and astrally.

Similarly, when you inhale the subtle aroma of lavender, the scent translates into the limbic system of the brain through the nose. This is the area which controls our emotions, consequently calming the patient and encouraging sleep. Bearing this information in mind, aromatherapy is what I consider a "wholeness assistant." It provides the body with extra tools with which to improve its own capacity for rejuvenation. While many people remain skeptical of such effects because of the lack of long-term testing, no one I know will dispute the benefits of a good massage or an aromatic restful bath!

Within aromatherapy, there are several approaches used. A clinical therapist works internally, prescribing small amounts of safe essential oils. Clinical aromatherapy should only be practiced by a trained professional. A holistic aromatherapist should be recognized by the IFA (International Federation of Aromatherapists). These people collect medical profiles and get an overall view of the patient's diet and lifestyle. They also consider the symptoms exhibited before deciding on the best aromatic applications and herbs.

Aromatherapy can be limited, however, to beauty treatments and general personal moods. This includes creams and lotions that benefit the skin, as well as herbal potpourri and perfumes that uplift the spirit. As long as you are not allergic to any scent chosen, and the oil is not known to have an adverse effect in concentrated quantities, then this form of aromatherapy is fairly safe to practice at home on yourself, on friends, or on loved ones.

Be forewarned, however, that essential oils can be very costly. If you are buying them, research available outlets first and find the most reasonable prices. Make sure the oils you purchase are in dark containers, and keep the bottles stored away from heat and light, which can be damaging. If you ever notice that an oil has taken on a cloudy look, this is a pretty good sign that its therapeutic effect is lost (the oil has gone bad from exposure to air and/or sunlight). Every oil has a different shelf-life, ranging from six months for citrus blends to nearly five years for resins and gums. In all instances, using a higher quality base oil for dilution will always extend longevity.

Aromatherapists also have some guiding rules-of-thumb for their profession. First, they know that the essences with which they work are highly concentrated. Therefore, more does not always mean better. Almost all essences have to be diluted before use, especially on sensitive skin. About the only exceptions here are lavender and tea-tree essences.

Second, essential oils need to be kept away from the eyes, as they can be very irritating and can even cause permanent damage. This is true even for inhalations. Third, when working with young children, *always* dilute the essential oils to one quarter of the adult potency for their protection. Lastly, always test any prepared oil on a small area of a patient's skin to be certain no allergic reactions result.

USING AROMATHERAPY

Please note that the way aromatherapists apply herbs will vary slightly. Included in Table 3 (page 63) are: inhalations, tonics, baths, nonaerosol sprays (which also work as air fresheners), and information about vaporization, medicine, massage, perfume, cooking, direct application, gargles, and compresses. WARNING: Under no circumstances should an essential oil be used to treat any condition on this list

Table 3. Herbs for Aromatherapy*	
HERB OR SCENT	APPLICATIONS
Aniseed	Indigestion, asthma, colds, cramps, stimulant, colic relief, stimulating milk flow, and insect repellant. May irritate sensitive skin.
Bergamot	Very versatile. Worry, tension, despondency, acne, itching, eczema, cold sores (especially if mixed with eucalyptus), throat and urinary tract infections. Do not use before being exposed to sunlight for elongated periods of time.
Caraway	Digestive problems. Use carefully.
Cedarwood	Externally applied for colds, specifically bronchitis; dandruff (mixed with rosemary), insect repellant, urinary infections, skin rashes. Not to be taken internally.
Chamomile	Resentment, change of life, menstrual problems, over sensitivity, anti-inflammatory, astringent, stomach ache, allergies, overall acceleration of healing process.
Cinnamon	Colds, warts, flu, joint problems, improved appetite, antiseptic quality. May be harsh on sensitive skin.
Citronella	Rheumatism, insomnia, headaches, insect repellant.
Clary	Throat problems, PMS, cramps, and melancholy.
Clove	Antiseptic, analgesic, toothache, indigestion, asthma. Makes an excellent toothpaste. Harsh on the skin in high concentrations.
Coriander	Weariness, indigestion, flu, agitation.
Cumin	Liver problems, headaches, stimulant.
Dill	General digestive difficulty, tension.

Table 3. Herbs for Aromatherapy (continued)

HERB OR SCENT	APPLICATIONS
Eucalyptus	Coughs, flu, joint and muscles, infections, expectorant, air freshener, mild antispasmodic, antiviral, fever treatment via compress. This is very strong; use sparingly.
Fennel	Digestion, nausea, weight control; ease constipation through back massage. Avoid use on sensitive skin.
Frankincense	Sleep disorders, phobias, anxiety, joint problems, fluid retention, comfort, decreased tension.
Geranium	Change of life, digestive trouble, balancing temperament.
Ginger	Aches, colds, digestion.
Grapefruit	Bitterness, stones, hardening of the arteries, despondency.
Hops	Sleep, bruises, cramps, tonic qualities.
Jasmine	Assurance, impotence, brooding, melancholy, introversion.
Juniper	Joints, cramping, menstrual regularity (baths), urinary problems. Pregnant women, or those suffering kidney infections should avoid this essence.
Lavender	Very safe. Burns, bug bites, skin disorders, sleep disorders.
Lemon	Colds, fever, cleansing qualities, astringent, general tonic.
Lime	Astringent, melancholy, gaining weight, insect repellant, headache.
Marjoram	Tension, high blood pressure, sleep disorders, stress, asthma.

Table 3. Herbs for Aromatherapy (continued)	
HERB OR SCENT	APPLICATIONS
Myrrh	Bacterial and fungal infections.
Nutmeg	Flu-like symptoms, overall aches, sleeplessness, joint problems. Not meant for long-term treatments. Pregnant women should avoid.
Orange	Tension, spasms, overall tonic, mild sedative.
Orange Blossom	Pressure, sleep disorders, immunity.
Oregano	Viral infections, especially colds. Digestion.
Patchouli	Acne and other skin inflammation, dandruff, insect repellant. Anti-fungal (combined with rosemary).
Peppermint	Stress (mental), memory, intestinal disorders, overall aches and pains, flu-like symptoms. Apply in minute quantities.
Pine	Bladder and kidney, chest infections, circulation. Be certain to use *pinus sylvestris* only.
Rose	Irascibility, disorientation, trauma, menstruation regulation.
Rose Geranium	Antiseptic, slows bleeding, skin treatments, harmony, mild sedative, insect repellant.
Rosemary	Memory, joints and muscles, circulation, stimulation and improved energy, digestion, dandruff, skin cleanser, susceptibility to sickness. Pregnant women should not use.
Rosewood	Tension, sleep disorders, cramps, digestive irregularity.
Sage	Bacterial infection, joint problems, astringent, swelling. Especially good mouth rinse for gingivitis (not to be swallowed). Do not use during pregnancy.

Table 3. Herbs for Aromatherapy (continued)

HERB OR SCENT	APPLICATIONS
Sandalwood	Anxiety, pressure, self-assurance, urinary problems, throat problems, colds, soothing dry skin. Improved self-confidence.
Spearmint	Cramps, digestive trouble, hemorrhoids.
Tea Tree	Joints, canker sores, burns, bug bites or stings. May be applied in undiluted form as antiseptic, antiviral, and antifungal.
Thyme	Joint problems, wounds, tonic, immunity improvement, bacterial infections. Always dilute before using; do not use on children or pregnant women.
Violet	Weight control, skin infections, analgesic, inflammation.
Ylang-Ylang	Hypertension, frigidity, ire, sadness, tonic.
Vetiver	Tension, nervousness, stress.

*Some affiliations used in this table are drawn from Robert Tisserand, *The Art of Aromatherapy* (Rochester, VT: Healing Arts Press, 1977). Most affiliations were common to many books on aromatherapy, but readers will probably want to explore these further.

without first consulting a complete guide to aromatherapy. Some oils, if used incorrectly, can be very harmful. Of all the oils listed, the safest and most commonly used in a personal aromatherapy kit are lavender, tea tree, peppermint, chamomile, eucalyptus, geranium, rosemary, thyme, lemon and clove.

HOMEMADE TOOL KIT

For the nonclinical aromatherapist, there are many aromatherapy preparations or methods that can be devised at home easily and inexpensively. Better yet, one need not be "into" aromatherapy to enjoy the results. Massage therapists, for example, might want to make their own scented oils, each of which is specifically geared to different effects. Acupressurists or reflexologists may choose to make an aromatic cream to keep their hands soft for work. Or homemakers may want to anoint their light bulbs with rose and lavender oil to renew love and peace in a tense home. Aromatherapy allows for a lot of creativity! Here are a few recipes and techniques to try.

Attar of Roses: One of the most valuable substances of all time, this is the pure oil of the rose, which is quite potent. If you have a rose bush at home, or have a friend who will allow some regular picking, you can get small amounts of this substance to use in your art. Roses are especially good for healing emotional wounds, and for engendering a renewed love of self.

Begin by picking only rose petals (no leaves or green parts) before 10:00 A.M. Simmer these slowly in warm water until they turn translucent. Squeeze the petals gently, then remove them from the pan (preferably nonaluminum). Finally, chill the water. After a little while, you will notice some small dots of what appears to be fat floating on the top of the liquid. This is rose oil. Store it in an airtight, dark jar, in a cool area and use small amounts as needed. This process sometimes works for other flowers too!

Scented Oils: Oils have a great number of applications, some of which might not immediately come to mind. Place a little on light bulbs to literally "light up" your mood with their scent. Use a lemon-based oil to condition wood and cleanse an area of negativity. Start with olive oil and add symbolic culinary herbs to fill your foods with metaphysical energy and indirectly, your home when those fragrances waft through the house while cooking!

Scented oils are incredibly easy to make, and teaching people the basic technique is equally simple. As a result, patients can start making their own aromatic blends to continue treatment when the therapist cannot. The only caution here is to accompany any such home efforts with specific instructions on what aromas to use, in what strength, and when.

To begin, choose your base oil. I suggest readily available cooking oils for anything that you want to be edible. Almond oil is also a wonderful base for all scented oils; it has a long shelf-life. Wheatgerm and avocado oils are nice as part of any skin preparation because of their high vitamin E content. Jojoba oil is excellent in massage blends, and sunflower and safflower oil tend to be good for any skin type.

Warm the oil, then add 1 tsp. of herb per cup of oil. For less aromatic herbs, you may need a little more, but take care that they aren't caustic to the skin. Mix and match your herbs for their desired effect, smelling regularly until you're happy with the aroma. Strain the oil and store in a dark, airtight container that is well labeled. This base can then be used in creams, sprays, and many other preparations.

As a side note, some people argue that oils made this way are not as potent as those that come from essential oils, which are then diluted. Since aromatherapy works on a vibrational level, I personally believe these homemade oils can be just as beneficial if made with loving care. Nonetheless, you should consider how you feel about the difference between a scented oil and a distilled or expressed aromatic, then decide what is best to accent your hands-on healing.[4]

---

[4]If you prefer high quality essential oils, write for catalogs from these two companies, both of whom I recommend highly:

Lotus Light/Blue Lotus
Box 1008
Silver Lake, WI 53170
Phone: 1-800-548-3824
Fax: 414-889-8591

Frontier Herbs
Box 299
Norway, IA 52318
Phone: 1-800-669-3275
Fax: 319-227-7966

Candles: You don't have to make candles from scratch to enjoy aromatherapy. Instead, light a candle, then add one or two drops of essential oil to the wax as it melts. Take care to keep the oil away from the flame.

Aromatic Bath: Add a maximum of 7 drops of oil to the tub and soak for about fifteen minutes. Look particularly to restful herbs. Thyme, rosemary, and marjoram are all good pantry choices.

Aromatic Fire: Add one or two drops to a log and let it age that way. Wood is porous, so it will continue absorbing the scent. Burn as desired.

Room Sprays: Use a small spray bottle, like those sold at garden shops for plants. Mix about 6 drops of oil to one cup of water. Shake before each use. May be applied anywhere that nasty odors hide. Citrus oils make especially fine room sprays, cleaning away the old and then reenergizing the area.

Light Bulbs: Two drops to a bulb is more than enough to scent an average-size room for several hours.

Tissues: If you have a special box that holds tissues, place one or two drops of oil in the bottom. Use those oils that promote health. The open weave of the tissue will naturally absorb the scent and encourage wellness for all who use them!

PERFORMING AROMATHERAPY MASSAGE

Before considering giving anyone an aromatherapy massage, check their physical condition. Those with heart disease, high fever, broken bones, skin disease, blood pressure abnormalities, nausea, and sunburn are not good candidates for a massage. You could do more harm than good. Additionally, be sure to ask about any allergies your patient may have.

With those precautions in mind, you next should evaluate what scent(s) are best for your patient. Wash your hands thoroughly, wear comfortable clothing, warm your hands and/or the oil before beginning, and remember to start out lightly. If someone wants a deeper massage, they'll say so.

Similarly, your subject should recently have taken a shower so their skin will accept the oils more readily. Make sure they're comfortable and warm; no amount of massage will help someone if they feel discomfort the entire time. Adjust the lighting in the room so it is soothing and open a bottle of scented oil so it can fill the room with an appropriate fragrance.

The floor is the best commonly available place for a massage as it does not "give" with your movements (as does a bed). Fold a couple of blankets and lay them out to provide some cushioning. Clear your mind of negative thoughts, and focus all your attention on the patient. Extend intuition with gentle strokes, changing oils if you feel it necessary.

Sometimes starting at the hands and feet helps relax both you and the patient. This is a good time to ask questions and just "chit-chat" a little. Once patients begin to relax, they will likely share information that you need.

Take your time, moving in smooth, even strokes at first, then focus on tension points. Be aware that not all your results here will be physical; some people may respond emotionally through giggles or crying, for example. For these people, the renewed flow of energy unblocks feelings that may have added to their problems and hindered real recuperation.

As with so many other healing arts, aromatherapy draws on a deep abiding respect for nature and its delicate workings. Not everything that is "natural" is good for the human condition. Similarly, just because something helps a problem, doesn't mean that the problem is necessarily cured. Aromatherapists must keep all this in mind as they serve, often sharing advice on other forms of alternative or traditional medicine to round out the patient's treatment.[5]

---

[5]For more general information on aromatherapy in the U.S.A., you may contact these associations:

American Alliance of Aromatherapy
Box 309
Depoe Bay, OR 97341
Phone: 1-800-809-9850
Fax: 1-800-809-9808

Aromatherapy Institute for Research
Box 2354
Fair Oaks, CA 95628
Phone: 916-965-7546
Fax: 916-962-3292

Pacific Institute of Aromatherapy
Box 6723
San Rafael, CA 94903
Phone: 415-479-9121
Seminars.

3

Auric Cleansing and Balancing

Light, that creative agent, the vibrations of
which are the movement and life of all things.
—Eliphas Lèvi

THE AURA HAS HAD MANY NAMES AND REPRESENTA-
tions throughout history. Included in this list are shining
raiments (Jesus), an envelope of light (St. Philip Neri),
crowns, the nimbus and aureole (halos), and the headdresses of Egyptians that depict energy emanations. Each of
these has significance to our study of healing. According to
Lewis Spence, an aura is "an emanation said to surround
human beings, chiefly encircling the head, and supposed
to proceed from the nervous system. It is described as a
cloud of light suffused with various colors. This is seen clair-
voyantly, being imperceptible to the physical sight." [1]

From the portraits of saints and gods which show lumi-
nescent light, we realize that some artists in history either
sensed or envisioned auric power with enough detail to
capture it on canvas. In the case of Egyptian headpieces, ar-
tisans gave physical form to the aura, thereby expressing a
spiritual principle. Those who wore the headdresses were

---

[1]Lewis Spence, *Encyclopedia of Occultism* (New York: Fireside/Simon and
Schuster, 1989), pp.50–51.

leaders and priests—individuals blessed by, and in close contact with, the gods.

Basically, the aura is a physical atmosphere that surrounds us. Within this atmosphere, particles of energy are suspended, rather like the particles suspended by the asteroid belt in our solar system. In this case, however, each individual is the central point from which the auric oval or egg extends. On the average, this extension measures two to three feet, appearing much like the bands of light in a rainbow and extending even below the feet.

Some individuals with extremely potent personalities will have far more drastic auras. These are the people whose energy arrives at a gathering fifteen minutes before they do. Such individuals are either very popular or very annoying. There is little middle ground when an aura is so extensive and intrusive. Conversely, the auras of newborns and animals tend to be snug, simple, and uncluttered, which is probably why people feel a strong affinity for both.

Auras gauge mental development, karma and other spiritual conditions, health, the higher self's communications, and emotions. They are external representations of our most intimate thoughts, bearing, and demeanor. According to Cabalism, each individual is concentrated in the center of this egg into a singular point of consciousness we call the ego. This is why an awareness of "personal space" is important for auric healers.

Until the 1950s, there was no certain way to prove or refute auric energy. Then, a Soviet husband-and-wife team generated a new form of photography that used spark generators, film, and organic matter to startling effect. This process became known as Kirlian photography, which allows people who are not clairvoyant by nature to view and interpret auric emanations.

Some of the studies in this field have given us tremendous insight into the importance of the aura in healing. For example, when a leaf is placed on the film plate, and one half of it is cut away, the leaf still photographs as if it were whole. This indicates that there is an electrical pattern to living things that the "body" remembers. This pattern is the shape of wholeness.

Additionally, in Orphic philosophy,[2] the greatest personal achievement comes when one breaks free of this egg, releasing the spirit to return to the Source.[3] So, treating the aura is akin to treating the soul itself; something to be done unobtrusively and with the utmost care.

AURIC SENSITIVITY

Before moving forward into using the aura as a diagnostic or healing tool, first one must develop a keen awareness of it. Some healers have a great natural sensitivity. For others, however, time and patience are required to truly comprehend the intricacies of individual auras through any one of the senses. As mentioned earlier, the development of auric awareness is very helpful to the healers' work. Thus, some simple exercises are provided here to help those who feel lacking in this area.

Exercise 1: Seeing Your Own Aura

Find a room where you can control the amount of light. Close the shades so that the room is dim, but you can still see reasonably well. Place a black cloth on a table before you, then put your hand about 2 inches above it.

Now, close your eyes for a moment and take three deep, cleansing breaths. When you open your eyes, don't look directly at your hand. The auric image comes through

---

[2]Manly P. Hall, *The Secret Teachings of All Ages* (Los Angeles, CA: Philosophical Research Society, 1977), pp. 20, 60.
[3]Among Oriental mystics, this is known as the *absolute* condition that returns the spirit to Nirvana.

peripheral vision, not direct gazing. Instead, let your gaze wander slightly so nothing in the room is totally clear. Pay particular attention to the region about ½ inch away from the edge of your hand.

Don't get discouraged if you don't see something right away. Close your eyes and breathe again, then try opening them just a crack. Give your eyes time to adjust to the low light. If nothing appears, check your other senses. Do you smell, taste, or hear something different than before? If you place your other hand near the first one, can you feel anything? Usually, one sense will respond most strongly.

Make a record of your experience, noting which sense seems most predominant to you. Repeat this exercise daily until you feel more confident and aware.

Exercise 2: Energy Lines

This is a fun exercise because it may be visualized or sensed. Get comfortable in a room prepared in the same way as in the first exercise. If it's easier for you, try using candlelight instead of dim outdoor lighting.

Ground yourself again with cleansing breaths, while placing the fingertips of both hands together. Don't open your eyes right away. Instead, feel the body heat generated between your hands. Focus your attention on that energy until your hands are almost hot. Now, slowly open your eyes, again not looking directly at the fingertips. Around the edges of your hands a slight glow should appear. There will be brighter light between the fingers where the aura overlaps.

Next, slowly separate your fingertips, taking them in opposite directions. Watch and feel the energy lines stretch between your hands like taffy. Maintain this contact as long as possible without breaking the lines. With practice, this exercise will help you connect with other people's auric energy in a more constructive manner.

Exercise 3: Seeing Other People's Auras

You will need a willing, interested partner for this exercise. Set up your room as before, finding one wall that has no decorations or knick-knacks to distract you. Additionally, it is best if the wall is black, grey or white so auric colors show up correctly.

Put a chair two to three feet in front of the wall. Your partner sits here. You stand or sit near the other end of the room with a gentle light source behind you (a candle, small lamp, or window). Follow the general methods given above for grounding and inner focus.

When you open your eyes, don't look at anything specific. Just direct your gaze toward the wall. See if there are any shades of color/light or clouds visible near your partner. Let your vision remain slightly blurry, as this will help the process.

If you do see something, continue observing that region and ask your partner to think of specific, personally significant moments in his or her life, allowing time to bring memories to the forefront and see if these thoughts create changes in aura. A happy memory will often reveal itself in pink wisps throughout the aura, for example. If this memory pertains to love or friendship, it may center over the heart chakra.

If several repetitions of this exercise prove fruitless, check your other senses again to see if they can provide any clues. Remember that spiritual "sight" is not dependent on just your eyes. The vibrations of auric colors may be sensed on different levels, levels that are more meaningful to each healer's perceptions.

Exercise 4: The Energy Ball

This exercise is designed to help you become more aware of other people's energy. It is also just plain fun.

Begin by facing your partner, who holds out both hands with the palms up, thumbs touching. You hold your hands (palm down) over your partner's in the same manner. By tilting your hands slightly near the outer edges, this creates a spherical empty space between both sets of hands.

Keep the distance between the hands constant at around 6 inches apart. Both you and your partner should close your eyes and focus on the energy between your hands, seeing it as a sphere of golden light (or another color agreed upon in advance). Next, open your eyes, keeping your vision unfocused as before. When you can both sense the ball of energy, move your hands apart very slowly and let that ball grow. Don't move much more than 1 inch at a time or you're likely to lose the sphere, rather like a soap bubble bursting.

The next step is tricky. Try passing the energy sphere back and forth to each other, always placing it on the palm of the hand. It will feel warm and tingly. When you get really good at this, you can actually use the energy sphere like a beach ball!

In terms of healing, sometimes I use this exercise with a person who is uneasy with a procedure. At some point during our "play time," I allow the ball to slip and burst over the area of need. The resulting energy spreads like a warm, yellow cocoon that usually results in a bad case of giggles.

THE AURIC BODY

Within the aura, there are subtle subdivisions to consider. These include the level of health, vitality, karma, character, and the spiritual nature itself. The karmic aura is always in flux, as every action and feeling we have affects the present and future karma of our lives. This is the action/reaction region where emotions evidence themselves, such as anger appearing in bright red lines pushing forcefully outward. Usually, counselors and care-givers care for this auric region (see chapter 1).

The next region is that of character, which is far more stable, having our present and past lives as its foundation. The color of this region is personality-dependent. All healers touch the character aura in some way because of the trust patients give to their physicians. The main chore of the healer at this level is simply to comfort and reassure. Character transformations are not part of this picture. Lasting personal change only comes through individual choice and fortitude, not manipulation.

The spiritual aura doesn't usually evidence itself unless this nature is the most powerful aspect of a person. In this instance, it appears startlingly bright with colors that go beyond words for description. Usually, the spiritual aura hovers *above* the physical aura, over an individual's head, but apart from the other emanations. Connection between the two only occurs when someone is in close contact with the higher self, or the Great Spirit.

Unless you are focused on spiritual wholeness, this domain probably won't affect your work. For healers who do serve the spirit, dark spots appearing in this region indicate a source of trouble that must somehow be resolved. This area deals with an individual's connection with the divine, their responsibilities, and their ability to acknowledge their own soul. Thus, the healer must proceed with care, knowing that the individual must recognize a need before this region can be mended.

Finally, the health aura is the one that healers deal with most directly. It has been described as an intricate network of energy lines connecting the body geometrically, rather like Ley lines on the Earth. When one of these strands is broken or mis-routed, dis-ease occurs.[4]

---

[4]Please note that when I use the term dis-ease, it refers to any resulting malady, from a simple ache to cancer.

The health aura extends 4 to 8 inches from the body (on average). In a healthy person, this aura should be symmetrical with no breaks or odd bulges. It has three distinct levels, beginning with a physical aura closest to the skin, a secondary etheric aura that can be disrupted by the physical, and the vital aura, which is nourishing and quite literally reflects "vitality." If we are tired, this level responds with dimness or by decreasing in size.

The vital aura holds the astral body and tends to have a pinkish hue. When the vital aura is pale, dark, or negligible, it often presages death, either literally or spiritually. A healer's work may affect the vital aura, depending on the severity of illness.

Additionally, the vital aura interacts with the next level of emanations—the mental. In this region, our thoughts and feelings may dramatically affect the process of diagnosis and healing. When patients take a placebo that they believe to be real medication that will help them, the vital and emotional aura may improve temporarily. If the malady was caused by an emotional problem, the sickness could disappear altogether!

COLOR, TEXTURE, SOUND, AND SMELL

People gifted in clairvoyance tell us that, beyond the light emanations that flow from our bodies, colors, textures and/or sounds also appear. Each of these indicates something specific to a knowledgeable reader. Below is a brief listing for your reference. Please note that these are generalizations only. While color has some universal symbolism, the way each person reacts to it can alter its manifestation in the auric envelope. Additionally, the background against which the person is viewed and the clothing worn can also change the way an auric color appears. Therefore, keep your instincts keen when making observations.

Color

Psychic vision is the most common way in which auras are perceived, especially when people stand against a dark, plain backdrop in neutral-toned clothing (see also Part II, chapter 4, "Color Therapy").

Blue

General: Devoted ideals, especially religious, peace, intuitive nature. Especially good for adding into the auric envelope to decrease trauma and soothe pain.

Dark blue: Not recommended in cases of shock. On the other hand, very effective for sleep disorders. As a ray, this indicates incoming information and knowledge. Psychics readily display this color.

Sky blue: A learning process, positive emotional health.

Turquoise: Insatiable scholarship, especially in esoteric matters.

Brown and Black

Brown: Selfishness or muddied thoughts; tumors and cancer sometimes show up as brown or black in the aura. Conversely, a rich, healthy brown indicates an affinity and deep respect for the planet.

Black: Blockage, sickness, dark paths, impending death (a null region), depression.[5]

Green

General: Return to health, growth in personality, hope, providence, manifestation, regeneration. Caution must be used with green in cancer treatments; it

---

[5]Edgar Cayce, in his pamphlet on auras (Association for Research & Enlightenment, 1945) recounted a time when he nearly stepped into an elevator where everyone seemed to lack auras. That elevator's cable broke, killing everyone aboard. This leaves some auric sensitives curious about the role of "fate" as expressed in our energy fields.

can actually increase cancerous cell growth, instead of healthy tissue.

Muddy green: Jealousy, critical opinions, sometimes falsehood.

Pastel green: Calm evolution, slow steady changes.

Sage green: Flexibility, tolerance.

Emerald green: Growth, empathy, kindness, well-being.

Pine green: Excellent for decreasing stress.

Gray and White

Gray: Bigotry, restrictiveness, intolerance, lack of imagination, despondency.

White: Protective, true beauty, clean energy.

Metallics

Silver: Cleansing, purity, the lunar nature. Events or situations of great immediate importance.

Gold: The solar, masculine self, fire and energy; most often evident in spheric energy and rays. An excellent all-purpose color for cleansing, repair, and bandaging. Also a good protective color.

Orange

General: Ambition, pride, and dignity; trauma or pain.

Orange is the balancing color between the mind and body. A hue indicating transitions.

Apricot: Sedative qualities, composing one's demeanor, helps balance other erratic energies.

Bright orange: Activity, stimulation.

Brown-orange: In the lower chakras, an indication of intestinal trouble. In other parts of the aura, it represents lethargy and repressed feelings.

Purples

General: Psychic or occult awareness. The spiritual nature. A high vibration that stimulates the third-eye chakra.

Violet: Controls cell growth, aids the processing of medication, eases fever and indigestion.

Red:

General: The physical, materialistic nature. Red stimulates energy, good for circulation and improving low blood pressure, but often an indicator of other problems.

Pink: Affectionate energy, unconditional love, friendship.

Bright red: Anger, force, power, and passion.

Deep red: Intensity or eroticism.

Yellow:

General: Creativity; high conscious functions; sometimes pale, unrefined shades indicate sickness.

Bright, Crisp: Concentration, logic.

Mustard: Shrewdness, dexterity.

Pastel: Higher reasoning.

Textures and Shapes

This ability is very similar to object reading. The texture and shape of an aura is usually communicated directly to the hands during healing, although visual impact can also occur. Outside this setting, auras may be experienced any time you're in close proximity to another person. Try extending your senses on a crowded elevator sometime and see what feedback you get!

Smooth: Peacefulness; a gentle nature, health.

Hard: Closed-minded, reclusive, muscle cramps, tumors.

Itchy: Nervousness, untruth, skin irritations.

Bumpy: Possible area of illness, a difficulty to overcome.

Soft: Flexibility and compassion, possible weak structures.

Static: Lack of understanding, miscommunication, nerve disorders.

Rough: Agitation, distraction, calcium or fat deposits.

Cold: Areas where circulation is impaired or, near the heart, possibly an aloof personality.

Hot: Areas where the body is focusing energy, frequently manifests near the vital organs.

Bulging: Area of tension or pain "pushing" out toward the senses. This may manifest before the problem becomes noticeable.

Jagged: Often an indication of anger or extreme emotion, especially when near the head or heart. Severe cuts and bone breaks. Hysteria.

Sticky: Insecurity, a clinging nature, sometimes the lack of honesty. Matters of personal hygiene. In terms of shape, this manifests as hooks or tendrils reaching into others' auras.

Prickly: Fear of intimacy. Areas of isolated, piercing pain, sometimes intrusive personality.

Distinct, well-defined edges moving outward: A willful, deliberate personality, sometimes stubborn.

Swirling inward: Brooding thoughts; if location specific, may indicate a problem area, especially when near a chakra.

Off-center: Emotional imbalance; too much right- or left-brain activity. Withdrawal.

Sounds

For those who can not see or feel auras, sometimes the sounds they hear in an altered state become an alternative indicator. This clamor is something heard with "spiritual" ears; it may be sensed in the same way a deaf person *feels* music. Technically, this is called clairaudience.

Rhythmic, steady: Order, balance, sound reasoning.
Intense or loud sounds: Energy, possibly frantic feelings, high blood pressure, sometimes violence (physical, or emotional).
Deep droning: Depression, lack of energy, sadness.
Light bells: Joy, self-satisfaction, return to wellness.
Hissing: Suspicion, jealousy, misrepresentation, internalization of feelings that leads to stress.
Melodic: Inner harmony, symmetrical aura, fitness.
Static: Someone tuning life out, inability to understand signals, communication disorders.

Smells

Next in the sequence of sensory input comes smell. Every healer has one sense that they respond to most strongly. This is the one that will guide them repeatedly in interpreting auras. People who are truly gifted perceive several levels of this information, thus providing a stronger basis for analysis. Therefore, it is always good for healers to develop all their senses as much as is personally and physically possible.

Sickly sweet: Dishonesty, manipulation. Physically, may indicate people that overindulge themselves.
After-rain fresh: Restful, relaxed individual with flowing auric energy. If they are recuperating, an excellent sign.
Strong bitter aroma: Withheld emotions, blockages, ulcers, stress. Often sarcastic and caustic.
Light florals: Sometimes the type of flower is significant here, like a rose fragrance from someone falling in love. Floral scents can also indicate the presence of a strong spirit guide. Usually indicative of joy and fulfillment.

Mold or must: Cancers, severe kidney infections, and many terminal illnesses carry this scent. The body is returning to the earth from whence it came.

Rich earth: Growth, new beginnings, strong ecological understandings, someone with good foundations. In folk medicine, good soil often buried sickness. This person is on the road to recovery.

Fruits: Like flowers, can vary according to type. However, in general, fruit aromas are positive indications emotionally and physically. It means an improved focus on one's diet, rest, and physical activity.

Greens: Like a garden after the rain. Incredibly refreshing. In healing, this is an indicator of renewed strength, improved outlooks, and active involvement toward wellness from the patient.

Spicy: Enthusiasm, energy, something's definitely cooking here! Just as the blend of spices makes or breaks a meal, whatever this person is doing is going to affect their auric field soon. For example, if the spices smell "hot," caution your patient to slow down a bit.

AURIC HEALING by Arawn Machia[6]

Auric work is very multidimensional. The more a healer develops all their senses, the more their diagnostic and healing ability will likewise improve. Also, if the healer chooses, they may add other tools to auric work like crystals and pendulums. These tools act like extra nails in the home-builder's kit by adding strength to an already well-devised technique.

---

[6]Used by permission. Arawn Machia is a psychologist, Reiki master, high priest in the Strega tradition of witchcraft, spiritual counselor, and well-respected national lecturer. He currently travels the country regularly, and is available for workshops. For more information, write, 1511 E. Commercial Blvd., #131, Ft. Lauderdale, FL 33334-5717. Please enclose a SASE.

One of the difficulties of auric work, however, is its intimacy. A patient must have confidence in their treatment, and learn the distinct difference between "sensual" and "sexual." For example, it's quite common for individuals to fall in love with their auric healer because this person performs a valuable, private service that deeply affects the patient's spirit. This is normal, but could be avoided with proper objectivity between patient and healer.

In all avenues of healing, but especially in auric work, attunement is essential. Many people don't realize just how naturally aware they are of spiritual energies. For example, go to the library and pick up a worn magazine then close your eyes. Try to picture the people who've handled that book, smell their perfumes, hear their whispers. The more you practice, the more exacting impressions become. Later, these impressions help the healer's art tremendously.

In terms of the aura itself, I must stress that there are no rules etched in stone to follow for diagnosis and relief. Each individual reacts to energy differently, and therefore evidences problems differently. One person expresses anger as a red energy exploding from their head, while another releases it from their heart, for example. Similarly, an itchy spot in two different people's auras does not indicate the same problem; it is simply a sensual manifestation—a cue that the healer must further define. Finally, externals can affect auric emanations too, so all these things have to be taken into account.

I learned how to interpret these cues as a child, so people shouldn't feel discouraged if they can't always get specific impressions in their first few years of practice. Also, if a healer feels the need to really prepare themselves before trying to sense the aura, this shouldn't make them feel like any less of a healer. Results are what count. A healer's job is to enhance life. If you achieve this in any degree, with or without elongated self-preparation, count your time and efforts as successful.

OTHER AURIC ELEMENTS

Besides the auric egg, there are other elements to our energy sphere reported regularly by clairvoyants and sensitives. Each individual perceives these slightly differently (by a feeling, scent, or inner vision). In the healer's work, recognizing these elements will decrease confusion over unique variances in energy, and can often direct the course of treatment more rapidly.

Rays

These are beams of energy that come from external sources to feed the chakras. They may come from loved ones or friends through their good wishes, thoughts, or prayers. They may come from guides, spirits, and teachers on other levels of existence, and also from the universe itself. No matter what the source, when rays intersect the aura, their location and intensity are important to the healer. They may provide vital clues to areas of need, or areas that are already being attended to.

Spheric Energy

Sometimes called "guide energy," this is a bundle of colored light located on one level of the aura in a specific location. As with rays, this bundle is accepted into our personal field to help with something specific on a conscious or subconscious level. Like an electrical outlet located on only one wall of a room, it supplies energy to a select region of the body, mind, or spirit if accepted by the host. The placement, movement, and overall character of these spheres may help diagnose less obvious problems.

Chakras

The predominant centers of energy that process both incoming and outgoing signals. Major chakras are located throughout the body (see list below). The degree to which any one center is open or closed (bright or dark) and what color they exhibit are all important factors in healing. The healer then must interpret these findings and channel the right energy for the right purpose.

Below is a listing of chakras and their associated maladies. Each individual examined can potentially feature sickness in the chakras differently. As a general trend, a healthy center exhibits clearly defined color and uniform light intensity. One that is only partially open, closed, or disrupted appears dimmer, muddy, lopsided, or splotchy.

Tailbone: Automated functions of the body, particularly the immune system. Also the spine and kidneys. Emotionally, this is the "fight or flee" instinct, compulsiveness or rigidity, and basic sexual drives.

Genital region: Perceptions and emotions, intestinal and digestive trouble, ulcers. On a minor level, nervous stomachs. Also aging disorders, reproductive problems, and the endocrine system. Chronic fatigue syndrome or hyperactivity.

Solar plexus: A personal power point filled with creative energy. Over-developed, this expresses itself as uncontrolled rage and ambition. Under-developed, it is fear and meekness. Physical manifestations include problems with the stomach, gall bladder, and liver.

Heart: The power of love, both in giving and receiving. If under-developed, the more animal instincts prevail. Over-developed, it expresses itself in a constant quest for love, companionship, and acceptance. Heart disease, circulatory distress, and asthma are associated with malfunctions of this chakra.

Throat: Thyroid, metabolism, bronchial trouble, stuttering, and weight problems. Emotionally, the throat chakra evidences our ability to communicate with others and ourselves. People unable to express themselves or who always hold their tongue may develop red spots in this chakra, indicating undeclared anger or important feelings.

Third Eye: Also called the agna[7] chakra, which I suspect may relate to a Latin term meaning *born in addition to.* This is the seat of mental and spiritual functions, specifically psychic insight. Disruptions here evidence outwardly as sleep disorders, hormonal imbalances, nerve problems, disorientation (possibly Alzheimer's), and general mental aggravation.

Crown: This center controls the flow of energy from the physical auric body to the spiritual. When blocked, people become despondent and troubled by life's meaning because they are not receiving "cosmic" energy from higher sources. The lower animal nature becomes primary. Chronic depression, resentment, antisocial tendencies, and lethargy may result. Physical representations: right-eye trouble, brain.

THE PROCESS

We can now look at the basic process of auric cleansing and balancing, using the aforementioned as a guide. The first step is becoming aware of the prevalent problems. The process healers use for their diagnoses differs slightly, but some commonalities did appear in my research.

Meditation and Visualization

In meditation and visualization, healers take time before they begin their work, envisioning the individual in their

---

[7]Joseph Ostrom, *You and Your Aura* (London: Aquarian Press, 1987), p. 51.

mind's-eye. As they do this, they begin to "feel out" the aura using their strongest sense. Some may actually envision the areas of difficulty as dark spots or tangles, while others perceive sickness as a smell, sound, or texture in the field. All of this is done without directly contacting the aura.

Pendulums

The pendulum is a simple device made with a cord or string attached securely to an object, frequently a crystal. Alternatively, some people use a favorite necklace. Generally a 6 inch length of cord is good.

To begin, healers hold the pendulum perfectly still, as close to one chakra center as possible without touching it. They then focus personal power, surrounding the pendulum to energize it. This interacts with the patient's aura, causing movement.

As the pendulum moves, healers observe its motion, rate, and direction. Areas where counterclockwise movement or no movement exists are centers that are either closed down or blocked. Elliptical movements toward the right or left indicate an imbalance of energy on the indicated side. Vertical swings indicate a strong focus on the spiritual, perhaps to excess, while horizontal swings denote blockages, especially in the emotions. Erratic movements are a sign of change in that energy center.

Hands

In perhaps the most prevalent form of direct diagnosis, healers scan the aura using the palms of their hands, collecting impressions as they go. No light visualization accompanies this particular technique, as it is a fact-finding mission versus one that channels energy to the patient. The feelings healers get along the way provide the first clues about what that patient may need.

For example, should the auric healer sense a hard or blackened region in an individuals' strong hand, it could mean several things. The darkness may indicate a physical block (like a blood clot) or other injury. Less literally, it might also signify someone who finds it difficult to reach out to others.

BALANCING THE AURA

Once the healer diagnoses the problem, the second step is to bring the auric envelope back to smooth, even levels. Any malady (emotional, physical, or spiritual) puts the entire auric egg out of symmetry. This irregular aura leaves patients feeling out of sorts, as if they were trying to walk all day in new shoes. The pattern they're used to has changed, bringing concurrent transformations in biorhythms.

It is interesting to note that health can also cause disruptions that manifest as an adjustment period. Usually this occurs with people who have been ill for long periods. Their bodies temporarily adjust to the imbalanced auric shell and then must readjust to the healthy energy.

Either way, using the rede, "as within, so without," as a foundation, healers know that balanced energy is an important part of the overall equation. Once they achieve this, the body's natural healing capacity and immune system function far better. Additionally, any other metaphysical efforts they make from this point forward will flow more smoothly.

I have seen some auric balancers use crystals for this part of their work. If you are interested in this approach, please read the chapter on crystal healing. The other major strategy is to pour gold or white light energy into the auric field like glitter. This energy is then smoothed into the aura as one frosts a cake.

The sensations this produces in the patient can be somewhat distracting to them. In *Hands of Light,* the author, Barbara Ann Brennan, explains this saying: "Most of us do not want our personal dynamics to be known by others. Most of us are ashamed of what will be seen if another human being looks closely."[8] Your aura, especially its inner levels, is very private. Healers should not violate or randomly intrude on that privacy. This is why auric balancers work slowly, usually beginning from the farthest level of the aura and working inward.

This approach provides the patient with an opportunity to integrate energy changes and become comfortable with the healer's technique. By the time the innermost layers are reached, the patient is open and prepared for that intimacy. From here, the healer continues to massage and adjust the aura until it is as close to symmetrical as possible, considering the patient's condition.

THE HEALING ACT

The third step is the healing act itself. For this procedure the palms are held downward over the inflicted area and the aura is massaged in a slow, circular fashion. Alternatively, some healers pull negative energy out of the aura with their hands (or a crystal) and then release it into the earth, the floor, or another neutral object. This is an important step for healers, so they don't accidentally "accept" the maladies of those they treat into their own auric energy.

At this point, touch therapy and massage may be added to the auric balancing to increase its effect. Clean energy, sometimes of a specific visualized color, is transmitted through the palms with loving care. This process con-

---

[8]Barbara Ann Brennan, *Hands of Light* (New York: Bantam, 1988), p. 59.

tinues until healers feel they have accomplished as much as possible.

Throughout the session, healers can instruct their patients on little ways to use similar techniques at home so they can become active participants in their own healing. Additionally, this approach to wellness can be repeated as needed without any ill effect for everything from tension relief to cancer. It should be noted, however, that this chapter has only provided a cursory overview of what can become a very technical process. I strongly encourage those interested in working with auric energies to read *Hands of Light,* an excellent resource with information useful to all practitioners of alternative medicine.

A Healing from Jackie

In 1984, Morgana was burned very badly in an automobile fire. Forty-five percent of her body had third-degree burns and the pain was excruciating. She didn't understand why the fire happened, and found a great deal of fear hindering her psychological healing, let alone her physical welfare.

Then she remembered the name of a psychic she'd met. Morgana's mother called Jackie and explained the problem. By the end of that week, this kind woman came to visit her in the hospital, fully prepared to psychically minister to Morgana.

Jackie shared some past-life impressions with Morgana, and also explained that she wanted to help ease her pain. Since Morgana's right thigh had hurt all week, despite conventional medicines, she agreed to the healing. Jackie explained that she approached healing very carefully, and that the pain Morgana felt would not extend beyond her wrist. Apparently Jackie used the visualization of a black cloth around her wrist to stop any negative energy from spilling over.

Jackie reached her hand to one to two inches above Morgana's leg and began to "draw out" the pain, actually appearing to pull an invisible substance from Morgana's aura. For the first time in two weeks, Morgana had no pain. At the moment, it was totally re-placed with amazement and appreciation.

Six years later, Morgana would start applying Jackie's technique in auric healings given to others (see chapter 1).

This story is beautiful because it shows again that healing is a legacy. One kind act can blossom outward to bless many other needful people, be it now or many years in the future.

4

Color Therapy

We weave with colors
all our own.
—John Greenleaf Whittier

ANCIENT EGYPTIANS USED SPECIFICALLY COLORED stones as amulets and colored some of their temples for healing. Pythagoras (6th century B.C.) taught the use of color to cure disease. An Islamic philosopher named Avicenna wrote the *Cannon of Medicine* in A.D. 1000, espousing color as both a diagnostic tool (in the skin, eyes, hair, and fingernails) and a remedial. In the late 1400s, Paracelsus repeated this theme by creating colorful cures in the form of charms, herbal blends, and elixirs.

These sources set the tone for all that would come in terms of color research and therapy today. In the 1700s, experiments began on plants to determine how colors affected their growth. The results were quite significant, with the long-ranging effects still being felt today. Now scientists apply this material to help people grow food in color-specialized greenhouses in regions with poor soil or harsh climates. In other words, they are rejuvenating the earth through color!

In the human sector, psychologists and behavior researchers have continued exploring the effect of color in physiological reactions and emotional response. The way humans react to color comes from several sources. First, there is an ancestral code that remembers specific symbols from our earliest days on this planet. Darkness was fearsome, bringing all manner of dangers. Conversely, a bright sun and clear sky brought the time to hunt, gather, and welcome relief from the night.

Repetition of these cycles became the earliest teachers of the race, showing when to seek safety. Adults taught this by example to their children and their children's children, until the information became a silent code resonating within the human frame. This instinct continues to shape our behaviors. Black remains a frightening color, especially to children, while yellow and blue are welcoming. Most people work during daylight hours and gather together in supportive units (families) by night.

A great modern example of how these latent codes affect us comes from contemporary changes in schedules. Anyone who has ever had to work the night shift will happily recount the difficulties of adjusting to daytime sleeping. This pattern isn't natural to our code; we are not nocturnal creatures. Thus, making that change disrupts biorhythms temporarily, until enough repetition occurs to incorporate the new cycle.

Decreased sunlight in the night-worker's life can cause depression, irritability, and lethargy. We now know that sunlight provides vitamin D and several other nutrients to our bodies. Additionally, people deprived of sunlight (especially children and women) often experience a sense of melancholy that they can't explain or shake. How often have you heard people remark that they have "spring fever" or "the winter blues?" All of these reactions may be linked indirectly to ancestral codes.

The second influence is experiential. If your mother always made you wear blue shirts, for example, you may have grown to deplore them. In this instance, blue symbolizes restrictions and limits. Alternatively, you may consider blue the color of nurturing and protection, recalling your mother's actions.

CHAKRA	BROWN/ SYMPTOM	GRAY/ SYMPTOM	TREATMENT
Crown	Too pensive	Careless	Vibrant yellow
Throat	Too conversive	Introspective	Violet and yellow
Heart	Unloving	Too empathetic	Turquoise and red
Solar Plexus	Anxiety	Conceited	Blue and green
Base	Listlessness	Hyperactive	Red and green

Table 4. Color Associations: Symptoms and Treatment.

This type of personal association is paramount to the healer's work, both personally and for the patient. Minor changes in ambiance can dramatically transform your procedures. If red makes your patient(s) nervous, keep that color out of the work area, even if you find it invigorating. Or, leave the color in a region where it is only in your line of sight. In this way, you can use your own positive associations with that hue as an aid, but not allow it to disrupt your patient's focus.

People react powerfully to color and light changes on both conscious and subconscious levels. We know this through the expression of colors in the auric field (see Part II, chapter 3) and by observation. Browns and grays, exhibiting themselves in chakra points, indicate the holding or blocking of energies, respectively. Once these colors are "seen" or sensed psychically, the healer can adjust by surrounding the patient with the appropriate treatment color, or by visualizing that hue filling the specified region (Table 4).

ADDING COLOR TO HEALING ROOMS

Have you ever noticed how many hospitals use green in their decor? This is a modern example of how color symbolism has reached far beyond New Age healing, into the physician's art. However, not everyone *likes* "hospital green." Therefore, we have to be a little more creative in our decorating schemes. Color does not have to be dramatic or intrusive in your personal space. Here are three examples that I've seen used effectively:

1. Have several sets of one-tone colored curtains. Put up the hue that best reflects the work to be done. As the light shines through the cloth, it disburses that wavelength vibration into the entire room! When you're finished, your traditional favorites can go back up!

2. Use colored lightbulbs. Similar in form and function to the curtains, these can be found at novelty shops or good lamp stores. An alternative is to save some of your decorations from Yule (like the candles) with different colored bulbs to use around your healing room. Again, once you complete the work, these are removable.

3. Knick-knacks, especially crystals, can gently reflect color and light into the room. Mirrors with watercolors on the surface are one example, along with stained glass window ornaments. Any small items can be placed neatly away, wrapped in cloth, between uses to protect them from unwanted energy.

This supportive tool kit can be added to any procedure without much fuss. It just takes a little forethought. Surround your patient with specially colored candles. Lay them on a piece of fabric or rug with specific hues or patterns. Add a bouquet of thematic flowers to the room, pieces of art, table accents, and furniture. In this way, every part of the healing environment reflects the needs of the patient and your personal vision. Following is a list of color correspondences for your reference:

Black: In terms of therapy, black is a collector for tension, and specifically, mourning. During the Victorian era, jet stone was favored as a charm to avert the sadness of loss. Black also symbolizes constancy and fortitude, the planet Saturn; its day is Saturday. If your patient is feeling at a loss, or needs to exert more tenacity, work with black as an accent color on Saturday for best results.

Blue: The celestial realms, gaining favor with spirits, and true wisdom are found in this color. Light blues represent peacefulness, the welcome calm after the storm, rest, and personal will. Dark blues pertain more to quiet and solitude. In India, statues and paintings portray Vishnu (and certain other gods) with blue skin to illustrate their divine disposition. In this philosophy, blue is the sacred color of the sun.[1]

Because it is a "water" color, this hue can act as a tonic on the entire system, reconciling energy that is out of balance. Light blue is commonly used by color therapists to treat throat problems, dark blue for the ears, nose, and eyes. Blue's planet is Venus, its day is Friday, and its number is six.

If your patient is suffering from the tensions of a rough relationship, place six blue stones over their heart chakra on Friday and guide them through a releasing meditation.

Brown: This is the earth, the soils of our land. Brown is a grounding color for foundations and fertile beginnings. It is also an apt color in which one may disburse negative

---

[1]Manley P. Hall, *Secret Teachings of All Ages* (Los Angeles, CA: Philosophical Research Society, 1997), p. 52.

energy of any sort. During warm months, take your patient to a comfortable plot of grass and direct their stress and sickness into the soil.

For individuals who have trouble keeping their heads out of the clouds, wearing brown or carrying a brown stone may help. This encourages the connection to Gaia.

Gold and Yellow: The Sun, the golden yellow of Leo, nobility, goodness, and creativity are found in these colors. Bright yellows speak of joy, zeal, and accomplishment. In ancient Rome, this was the hue of fertility and happiness. Consequently, yellow is an excellent choice for healing depression.

Gold reflects noble efforts and leadership as pure as the Sun god. If someone has self-doubts or cluttered thoughts, adding gold into their wardrobe won't hurt. In terms of physical health, yellow and gold relate to liver problems and skin disease.

Green: Order and cycles (note nature), growth and evolution. Green's day is Wednesday, and its planet is Mercury (for change). Emotionally, light greens encourage the sprouting of new ideas or characteristics. Lush, dark greens bring maturity and continued abundance.

During the 3rd century B.C., Theophrastus recommended green stones for eye trouble. This application for green stones continued through the Middle Ages. Directing this energy in a metaphysical setting, use a green stone on your third eye to become more open to psychic insights. Physically, green is recommended for heart disease and regulating blood pressure.

Purple or Violet: The spiritual nature, leadership roles (note royalty), and effective communication especially on esoteric matters. Violet is the color of good judgement and religious thought. Its planet is Jupiter and its strongest day is Thursday.

In terms of health, violet should be added to the rooms of those with sleep or nerve disorders. It has a calm, soothing effect that will help decrease tension and improve rest. It also can relieve headaches.

Silver and White: The Moon, contemplation, meditation, and the intuitive self. This is a cleansing, pure ray that brings victory over self-produced problems, especially your own emotions. Its day is Monday (Moon day) and its number is seven.

In Greece, Italy, and Rome, white was the color of mourning. It was also, interestingly enough, the hue of beginnings, faith, and purity. In concert, these meanings have tremendous power if one is trying to "kill" a bad habit or addiction.

Red: Energy, fire, assertiveness, conscious movement, heated emotions, drastic change, and power. In subtler shades, kind feelings and friendship. Red's day is Sunday and its number is nine. Within this pigment are the attributes of pride, command, leadership, and passion.

In healing, red is often used to increase personal energy and improve circulation (or help other blood-related difficulties). This is based upon the principle of similarity and sympathy (like producing like).[2] Emotionally, red can engender increased ability to love or take control in difficult circumstances.

THE SHAPE OF COLOR

The logical half of human nature yearns for form and order. Since a color therapist hopes to integrate conscious

---

[2]George F. Kunz, *Curious Lore of Precious Stones* (New York: Dover Publications, 1913), p. 370.

awareness of color and its effect into the patient's life, they will sometimes use colors presented in specific shapes to accent the effect. For example, a green pillar candle helps engender a feeling of balance and equilibrium. A red circle draws pointed attention, whereas a red square inspires active energy.

Exactly how color therapists apply this knowledge is pretty open-ended. They may instruct a patient to visualize the light-color of a meditation coming to them in a specific shape, or as having their bodies surrounded by a crystal of a suitable shape and color. Basically, adding shape to color therapy gives it an extra dimension that empowers the procedure. Here's a list of basic shape correspondences:

Circle: Feminine, lunar or solar (color dependent), completion, cycles;

Square: Foundations, masculine, guidelines, regulation;

Triangle: Fire, masculine, recognition, conscious awareness;

Diamond: Feminine, the womb, lunar, fruitfulness, intuitive;

Octahedron: Air element, sound, dreams, creativity;

Dodecahedron: Spirit, touch, deeper mysteries and truths;

Star: Attainment, renewal, rebirth.

APPLIED COLOR THERAPY

I personally believe color therapy is most effective when combined with other techniques. It is so easy to add it to nearly any approach to wellness. However, if you wish to use strictly color as your medium, you can consider the examples already given herein or those provided below.

The idea is to regularly bring one color or a combination of shades into the auric field of your patient until the light field returns to balance. Sometimes it is necessary to extend this effort into the home so that a continuing resonance of positive energy surrounds them. In this case, give your patient some of the hints that healers use in their workrooms for similar results.

Color Therapy Approaches

The easiest form of color therapy is through clothing and jewelry accents. The old saying, "clothes make the man," came about for a good reason. What we wear makes us feel and act differently. People who are depressed often don dark or neutral colors without thought. This only reinforces that emotion outwardly. Conversely, outgoing and happy people frequently wear bright, crisp colors reflecting their mental state.

Whatever the emotional or physical conditions, your job is to choose appropriate color(s) for each individual's well-being. If some are uncomfortable with wearing colors they don't like, try the crystal-carrying approach instead. Both techniques help produce the same effect, but the patient needs to feel comfortable with the choice of programs for best results.

Timing and Balance

Looking at, or surrounding yourself with, a specific color for a certain number of hours or minutes within a set cycle (day, month, week). Babies who have bright, well-lit rooms evidence more energy. As adults, we don't notice this change in ourselves because we're taught to maintain a certain outward image. However, the amount of light/color we receive every day does affect us.

In color therapy, you teach your patient how to balance out various spectrum deficiencies and excesses. People who stare at computer screens all day may find that the normal peacefulness of blue turns to lethargy or apathy after eight hours. They need an infusion of red or yellow to balance that saturation. Similarly, people who work in a production plant surrounded by silver tones and with little daylight may discover their thoughts wandering. For them, a goldtone or sunlight infusion at the end of the day is just what the "doctor" ordered!

As always, make sure you consider individual feelings about specific colors before deciding on a course of treatment.

Body Paint

An unusual and creative application for the color therapist. Think in terms of the Native American sand paintings, only on the physical body. Here, healers apply the vibration of color directly (nontoxically) to the skin in symbolic, empowering patterns. Then, when the paints are rinsed off, individuals may also envision their sickness (or their problem) being washed away.

Guided Color Visualizations

Most healers have specific visualizations that they use repeatedly, with minor variations, according to individual needs. Sometimes they combine these with appropriate music, like soft chimes for purple or upbeat drumming for red. Another accent is specially prepared incense that reflects the color's element, like pine for green or lily for blue. Each of these additions increases the subconscious impact of the visualization by harmonic reinforcement.

Four examples of guided visualizations follow. This is by no means a complete list of forms. Instead, these were assembled from the commonalities discovered during the research and interview process.

The first example involves instructing the patient to imagine colored light pouring down from the heavens. This imagery is easy for most people because it reminds them of the noonday sun, something familiar and welcoming. From here, the light either flows through the individual or pours over them like a waterfall, to interact with the aura.

The second type uses the colored sphere. This is especially effective for people who are frightened or feel insecure, as the colored light acts as a buffer. For this exercise, patients imagine themselves inside something akin to a soap bubble that is filled with colored light. This light is then absorbed into every pore, like water effortlessly flowing between grains of soil.

In the third type, the patient envisions colored light as the essence of air itself. In this visualization, the patient breathes in that color to incorporate its positive effects, then exhales any negativity. This imagery continues in a cyclical manner until the healer senses a maximum effect has been achieved.

The fourth example involves the visualization of a colored symbol or shape. The emblem chosen should be easily remembered and one that is a positive affirmation of what the patient needs. For muscular weakness, a healer might guide the patient to see a blazing red rune of the warrior (↑) to encourage strength. In this instance, the token and its color work together to increase the technique's impact.

Crystals and Light

An interesting adaptation of color therapy came to me through an artist in Florida. She has devised a way to integrate crystals into wands so that, as light shines through one end, it illuminates the other end with one or several colors. The overall effect is very beautiful, but also holds potential in the field of color therapy. For example, a crystal could be placed atop a light table to illuminate its facets and send those vibrations throughout the room.

Colored Oils

For a massage therapist, this is a really interesting option. Plants have natural colors that frequently express themselves into an oil medium without any difficulty. For instructions on how to make homemade oils, refer to the chapter on aromatherapy.

The Pigment Diet

Another unique, and usually fun, exploration of color therapy comes from foods and beverages. During the Middle Ages (and earlier) the idea of natural sympathy evidenced itself in the way various plants were used in healing. The belief was that God gave specific clues to treating the human body through the colors of nature. Therefore yellow roots or flowers were prescribed to cure jaundice. The pigment diet builds on this idea, balancing modern knowledge of toxicity with the symbolic content of the items suggested.

The pigment diet works exactly as it sounds: by adding more foods of a specific color to regular meals to effect results. For improved energy, consider adding red peppers. Since peppers have a cleansing effect on the system, the elimination of toxins may indeed improve energy levels! Alternatively, the idea of "growing" vitality could be accented with green spinach and other leafy vegetables. Dieticians will happily assert the value of these foods for raising iron levels that can dramatically affect physical stamina.

Here is a brief list of foods to consider for their colorful symbolism. Please note that the food's own symbolic nature combines with the color for its application in the therapy. Using red for an example, add apples to your daily diet to encourage physical energy for well-being and continued health.

Red: Pink grapefruit (purification), apples (health), strawberries or raspberries (joy), tomatoes (love).

Yellow: Bananas (sex), yellow grapefruit (cleansing), lemon (fidelity), yellow beans (prosperity), honey (health and communication).

Orange: Oranges (health, fidelity), yams (the divine nature), carrots (vision).

White: Chicken breast (health), bread (foundations, providence, life), potatoes (grounding), onions (baldness).

Brown: Beef (prosperity), rice (providence, health), beans (oracles).

Purple: Beets or turnips (foundations or passion), red cabbage (any lunar-related efforts), blackberries (happiness).

Any color that is difficult to find in foods can be added to clear beverages via natural food coloring. For peaceful joy, add a drop of blue food coloring to sparkling water. For zestful energy, add a drop of red to ginger ale! Get creative and provide your patients with easy, memorable ways to return to health.

5

Counseling

We give advice, but we do not inspire conduct
—Francois, Duc de la Rochefoucauld

COUNSELING AS AN ART IS FUNDAMENTAL TO ALL alternative healing methods. We must be good listeners to be good diagnosticians. We must also understand the fundamental differences between patients to be effective in our art.

Counselors give emotional or situational support and guidance that may or may not have anything to do with physical health. Nonetheless, psychologists agree that mental states can drastically affect the body, stress being one of the best examples to which almost anyone can relate.

Several attributes are necessary to being an effective counselor. They include:

1. Compassion;

2. The ability to separate yourself from the situation for objectivity;

3. Understanding how different personality types react to stimuli;

4. Understanding the short-term and long-term effects of social, emotional, and physical environments on personality and development;

5. Clear, concise communication skills.

In discussing counseling and the attributes of a good spiritual counselor with Arawn Machia (see Part II, chapter 3, "Auric Cleansing and Balancing"), he had these insights to share:

COUNSELING by Arawn Machia[1]

Spiritual counselors have a talent that responds directly to need and universal purpose. Their task is not an easy one. They must be nonjudgmental listeners, able to balance objectivity with a caring demeanor. Counselors must also be honest and loving throughout any session: honesty belays "wishy-washy" attitudes, and love offsets overly critical attitudes.

Additionally, counselors must think globally, recognizing that emotional stress evidences itself in physiological symptoms. The best way to achieve this focus is by remaining really open to Spirit, and by trusting their own ability to see beyond surface reality. A good counselor gets to the core of a matter, not just the trappings. At this juncture, a counselor's job also becomes one of education or re-education so that a patient realizes that everything is a matter of personal choice. What one chooses to think, to say, to do . . . this affects every portion of living.

Finally, at the end of a session, it is vitally important that integration occur. If a patient doesn't understand what's happened, the residual uncertainty can lead to depression. Depression then may lower immunity, opening the door for sickness, leaving the patient with two problems instead of one with which to cope.

[1]Material used by permission. See also footnote 6, p. 85.

During integration, a patient should be encouraged to ask questions and talk about what they see as the results of a session. Also, at this time, clearly defined goals should be set for the next meeting and the time between sessions. This helps leave people with a real sense of purpose, which leads to more assured action and longer lasting results.

From reading this, it is evident that counseling focuses on an exchange of ideas and opinions so that patients develop enough confidence to make their own decisions. Wellness is, indeed, a decision; being whole in mind and spirit is a decision. Each patient must resolve to live as contentedly as possible, considering the circumstances. The counselor's job is to help patients discern exactly how to achieve this goal.

The approach for each patient must be different for true success. Attempts at change can result in emotional scars if counselors do not understand the underlying motivations for, and personality type of, their patients.[2] After all, a declawed lion is still a lion, but, without that defensive mechanism, the lion becomes susceptible to predatory attacks. Similarly, one can not take the "fire" out of aggressive people without dampening their drive. Counselors must recognize this delicate internal balance and respond accordingly.

Making matters slightly more complicated is the fact that personal change is not an isolated thing. Our situations and the people around us can affect our search for wholeness in dramatic ways. Therefore, a good counselor reveals how different people can interact positively with,

---

[2]David Keirsey and Marilyn Bates, *Please Understand Me* (Del Mar, CA: Prometheus Nemesis Books, 1978), p. 2. This is an excellent self-study book that I recommend to anyone wanting to do a little introspection. It also details many personality types which will help all counseling efforts.

and learn from, each other through various exercises and free-flowing discussions.

Here is one example where "Jeff" is complaining of digestive disorders that seem to have no medical cause. The counselor takes time to gather his history, discuss his job, and go over the prevalent people with whom he interacts. We are entering the conversation halfway through a session to discover how the counselor helps Jeff discover the core of his problem.

Counseling Session[3]

Counselor: When do you find your stomach is most upset—after eating spicy foods, when you're around certain people . . . ?

Jeff: Never really thought about it. Spices don't seem to bother me much. I eat mostly with my family.

Counselor: Do you feel happy with your family? Are they happy with you?

Jeff: Basically. My aunt's a little pushy about her religion. Dad's a good hearted person, sometimes too much so, but he's pretty supportive. My sister . . . well, she's a little sister . . . you know.

Counselor: Do either your aunt's or your sister's actions bother you? Do they make you angry?

Jeff: Sometimes.

---

[3]This is a reenactment based on an actual situation. The gist of the conversation was relayed to me without revealing any names, so that the patient and healer could remain anonymous.

Counselor: Why?

Jeff: Because they don't seem to care about anyone else's feelings or ideas. It's as if they're the center of the universe.

Counselor: Would you say their statements or actions toward you or others you care about are sometimes hurtful?

Jeff: Yes.

Counselor: Do you try to do anything about these times?

Jeff: I used to, but that only made things worse. My aunt would take out her anger toward me on Dad, and my sister got more spiteful, so I just shut up or try and get out of the house.

Counselor: Is it possible that your stomach problems started when you stopped voicing what you deem "righteous anger?"

Jeff: Yeah, actually . . . I mean, you think that's the cause?

Counselor: What I think isn't important here. If you believe that's the cause of your sickness, we can try and find a good solution together. Otherwise, we'll keep hunting until we do find the source.

Jeff: No, I really think you're on the right track. I get so angry that everything knots up inside. I get even angrier because I *let* them bother me so much!

Counselor: Jeff, these are people you care about. Their opinions and actions are going to affect you—that's only human nature. Don't berate yourself for being normal. How do you think your reactions affect you spiritually?

Jeff: I guess it might make me more closed off. I don't want to be around people when I feel pissy.

Counselor: Do you use your anger like a shield? If so, what does it keep in and who does it keep out?

Jeff: You ask tough questions. I'll have to think about that for a while, ok?

Counselor: Yes, that's fine. You don't have to solve all your life's mysteries in one day, you know! By the way, do you have any physical outside activities right now?

Jeff: Not really, unless you consider going to movies and visiting friends "physical."

Counselor: Then may I suggest starting an exercise program or some other type of outlet you'd enjoy? This way you can work out your frustrations before eating—exercise will also help you digest food more efficiently. If you're willing to try it for a couple of weeks and make notes of your experiences, we can determine if this approach will work for you. We'll also keep meeting during this period.

Jeff agreed to give it a try. Since it was summer, he took to biking to and from work. As he rode, he visualized all the anger pouring into his legs, then being pumped out with every leg stroke. By the end of one month, except for minor irritation, Jeff's stomach problems were all but gone.

This example effectively illustrates how the counselor never made any decisions for the patient or attempted to coerce him into a specific conclusion. Instead, the conversation always returned to Jeff in the form of a question to encourage self-examination and analysis.

Finally, the counselor suggested a positive activity for Jeff that would help him control his emotions. Since Jeff could not get away from the situation causing the problem, he had to find a project that redirected his negativity. Each step of the way, Jeff remained an active, aware participant in making himself better.

PERSONALITY TYPES[4]

Understanding personality types and how they react (or interact) is the most important part of counseling, next to being an active, informed listener. Each type acts as a system of roots, giving form and foundation to a wholly unique tree. Since the source of dis-ease can potentially come from tangled or unhealthy root systems, we must begin our search here.

In reviewing these types, it is important to remember that very few people are stereotypical or strictly of one type. We all have small facets of different categories that affect the way we walk through this world. Anticipating just how much other facets affect the whole is a very difficult part of counseling.

Extraverts

Extraverts get energy from being with people. Sociability is central to the core of their self-worth; it is their power source. Extraverts feel terribly lonely when excluded from such activities. If they are forced into solitude for a long period, depression and chronic fatigue may result.

On the other hand, extraverts sometimes have trouble taking necessary time for themselves. They get caught up in social momentum to the point of speeding headlong into disastrous situations. When weariness increases, it leaves them more susceptible to colds, viruses, and other maladies

---

[4]These types are taken, with minor adjustments, from C. G. Jung's writings. Jung believed that everyone has fundamental differences. Conversely, he also felt that all people have central drives in common. The differences manifest because of the way people incorporate those drives into themselves, and how they exhibit that preference outwardly. To explore these psychological types further, a good introductory volume might be *The Portable Jung,* Joseph Campbell, ed. (New York: Viking, 1971), pp. 178ff.

caught from contact. In the most serious cases, people can give themselves ulcers and other stress-related conditions because they don't know how (or when) to stop. The challenge to counselors here is to teach their patients that being alone does not necessarily equal loneliness, and that periodic retreats are healthy.

Introverts

Introverts are territorial. Personal space, privacy, and quiet are essential to introverts' well-being. They feel uncomfortable in crowds to the point of isolation. In fact, introverts are exhausted by contact and need regular breaks to cope with social interaction.

Introverts have generally fared less well in society than extroverts. Frequently people criticize them for being too reclusive or stand-offish, misinterpreting their behavior as snobbish. The most difficult thing for introverts to learn is that they do not have to feel guilty for needing "down time." Instead, they must make others aware of this need so it is understood and respected—a difficult task for people who aren't overly at ease with intimate communications.

If introverts don't get enough personal time, they begin exhibiting tension, anger, worry, and nervousness, seemingly over nothing. They may seem to drag their feet and lack motivation. When they come home at night, they might turn into chronic couch potatoes in an attempt to reclaim some isolation. In worst-case scenarios, they become paranoid and overreactive. These individuals need private vacations badly. Get them away from everything, if only for a few hours, so they can recharge their batteries.

Sensibles

These people are detail-oriented. Experience and history are of ultimate importance to sensibles, who seek *reality*, not fiction. Sensibles base decisions on what they consider to be sound reasoning; they want no part of nonsense, flights of fancy, or gut instincts.

Sensible personalities make great number crunchers, but find it hard to believe in their dreams. These are difficult people to work with spiritually, because spirituality can not be proven in black and white. They can also be fooled by appearances, because intuitive feelings get pushed aside as useless—as feelings are not *facts*.

When sensibles' perceptions deceive them, it can lead to bitterness and sometimes violence. When people wear the sensible blinder, they believe the rules of reality should not change. When the rules do change, it causes confusion and strong pangs of remorse. They can not understand how logic failed them. For these individuals, learning that we live in an illogical, disorderly world is the greatest coping mechanism. It relieves some of the self-generated pressure to be 100 percent correct all of the time.

Intuitives

Someone with an intuitive nature depends on imagery, metaphors, and symbols. For an intuitive personality, the imagination is a tremendous tool through which all kinds of possibilities can be explored. These people believe wholeheartedly that every door has a key—it just has to be discovered. Intuitives are always planning for tomorrow, basing those plans on hunches and hopes, but not always completing them.

Jung described intuitives as individuals who plant their gardens, then race off toward new adventures without waiting to see those seeds come to fruition. Since today is only a way-station for these people, they can become overly fidgety and disappointed when reality doesn't measure up to their dreams.

Additionally, intuitives are also more susceptible to "New Age" gimmicks, wanting desperately to experience the sublime world. These individuals need an anchor to the Earth that offers enough slack for creativity, but enough discipline to avoid hoaxes.

Thinking

These people make decisions based on logic. They look to rules and objectivity to guide them. They are often regarded by others as being somewhat distant or emotionally cool, because they don't like exhibiting their feelings. Thinking people make great debaters, always wanting to anticipate both sides of a question. However, they rarely let their hearts rule their heads, and therefore sometimes miss out on spontaneous pleasures.

Feeling

Feeling people dislike "carved in stone" ultimatums. For them, personal impact and values are essential to the human equation. These individuals tend toward romantic idealism and softheartedness, even when its not in their best interests. Feeling people will often have trouble standing up for themselves and will avoid arguments, if possible. Therefore they make excellent caregivers, but are frequently taken advantage of until they find their "fighting spirit."

Judgmental

These individuals want closure in their lives. Everything needs to be certain and concrete. If a decision is to be made, they urgently try to do so within a deadline. They constantly check watches, plan their time, organize, and have an amazingly strong work ethic that can easily turn into work-a-holism. Judgmental personalities think in terms of necessity; they will do whatever it takes to get a job done, even if it means self-sacrifice.

Persons in this category have contagious drive, but may appear inflexible and pressure-oriented to outsiders. Unfortunately, because of the compulsive tendencies latent in this personality type, many of them overdo, resulting in heart attacks, ulcers, sleep disorders, and difficulty maintaining any relationships that don't somehow interact with their goals.

Perceiving

Perceiving people resist finalities. They always prefer to keep their options open and fluid. When given a stricture, like a deadline, perceiving individuals may give themselves an *earlier* goal date, just to keep a margin of a few days or hours to accomodate minor changes or disruptions.

In terms of decision making, these individuals want as much information and as many selections as possible (which often delays everything). On a more positive note, they tend to evidence the inner-child more freely, and thus are more open to metaphysical information and experiences.

There is much more that could be written about personality types and their effect on counseling, but space prohibits such a lengthy discussion. Being a spiritual counselor is not necessarily something that requires schooling and lengthy study, but understanding personality types is a good place to begin. Additionally, take a cue from the greatest counselors of history by learning to perceive, hear, creatively question, and gently guide those who seek your aid. As I mentioned earlier, sometimes the greatest gift of healing is nothing spiritual whatsoever, but the willingness to be there, listen, and care.

6

Crystal Healing

Behold, I will lay thy stones with fair colors and lay the foundations
with sapphires. And I will make thy windows of agates, and
thy gates of carbuncles and all the borders of pleasant stones.
—Isaiah 54:11, 12

THE ANCIENTS LOVED GEMSTONES. THERE IS AN abundance of superstition surrounding them. From the Egyptian paintings to the writings of the Victorian era, history indicates that gemstones were used in everything from making wishes to protecting people from the evil eye. What was it that captured humankind's interest with such ferocity?

At first, it was likely the simple beauty of stones that attracted our attention. In the case of luminous stones, animistic peoples credited them with having indwelling spirits that could be appeased for favors. Thus, simple folk beliefs gave birth to the first good-luck charms!

Gemstones also appeared in the writings and practices of various religious groups. The Egyptians wrote sections of the Book of the Dead on semiprecious stones as a kind of prayer or invocation to protect their departed ancestors.[1] In ceremonial worship, Hindus recognize many offerings

---

[1]George F. Kunz, *Curious Lore of Precious Stones* (New York: Dover Publications, 1913), p. 225.

which include gems and jewelry. The Navajo's depict rain-making gods with necklaces of coral and turquoise. And, the Old Testament (Exodus) describes a breastplate worn by Aaron and the subsequent High Priests of Israel bearing twelve stones, one for each tribe. These examples only begin to explore the broad-ranging use of stones in the religious worship of the ancients.

During the 1100s, St. Hildegard, the abbess of a Benedictine nunnery, wrote about crystals and their effectiveness for managing disease. She believed that their brilliance reminded Satan of his former glory. This painful truth being too much for evil to bear, makes Satan and his minions flee from the light. By using this philosophy, a patient vexed by the demons who manifest illness could benefit greatly by using crystals regularly. Some of St. Hildegard's prescriptions included lapis for eye trouble, jasper for hearing, diamonds for jaundice, and chalcedony for gall bladder difficulties. At least some of her teachings had long-lasting effect. In 1531, for example, Pope Clement VII drank large quantities of powdered gemstone for his own recovery, at substantial expense.

Later, alchemists and philosophers considered gemstones in a slightly different light. Crystals are formed by the land, come from the soil, absorb energy from the planet, Sun, and celestial realms. They reflect the amazing power of Gaia, once unearthed. Thus, the older the crystal, the more potent it's likely to be, at least in theory. This, along with their hardness, is perhaps why the ancients revered diamonds so highly. For a while, people even drank diamond dust to cure certain diseases![2]

Diamonds were not the only gem to acquire such unique meaning. Nearly every precious and semiprecious stone on this planet has been used as an amulet, charm or talisman, most usually in the form of jewelry. It is particu-

---

[2]Clusius, *Aromatum Historia* (1579), quoted in George Kunz, *Curious Lore of Precious Stones* (New York: Dover, 1913), p. 153.

larly interesting to notice where people chose to place their adornments: on the wrist, ankle, and neckline (near pulse points); on the forehead (near the third eye or spiritual center); over the heart chakra (our emotional center); off the waist (near the center of gravity). These placements were not accidental, and hold import for crystal-healing methods today.

Consider your spiritual body for a moment as a huge fuse box from which hundreds of circuits radiate throughout your body and aura. These lines carry energy and signals, both good and bad. When you hurt, they convey the pain. When you're happy, that emotion flows and evidences itself in physical changes—a smile, a more positive stature, perhaps even jumping.

Carrying this idea one step further, crystals also have a basic matrix that can house or transport energy (notably quartz and coal). When this natural indwelling power reacts with our own auric field, some changes are likely to result. In *Crystal Secrets* by Brett Bravo,[3] the author calls this the "tuning fork" effect, where two items begin to vibrate on the same frequency to maintain harmony. Bravo also recommends adding personal thought forms transmitted through the crystal to amplify healthful effects. This basic formula is a fairly universal description of crystal healing.

CRYSTAL CLEAR

The best part about crystal healing is that, like auric work, Earth healing, color therapy, aromatherapy, and other subtle arts, it is something easily learned and incorporated by anyone. If you bring a piece of earth into your home, even if your choice was "wrong" for an ailment, it certainly won't

---

[3]Brett Bravo, *Crystal Healing Secrets* (New York: Warner Books, 1988), p. 7.

hurt you. By the effort you have at least acknowledged nature's ability to aid in healing—an action whose power is not to be underestimated.

Additionally, because of the popularity of crystals, no one will think you odd for having a few pretty "knick knacks" around the house! So, if Aunt Sadie visits regularly but regards alternative medicine with disdain, your newly acquired talent need not even come up in conversation. I don't advocate hiding behind such guises often, but, because we still live among people who do not adapt to change readily, there are moments when having a little camouflage decreases social stress considerably.

CHOOSING CRYSTALS

Exactly which crystals are chosen for an illness depends on several things, including color symbolism. Thus the study of color therapy and crystal healing cannot be totally separated. Additionally, the natural makeup of the crystal, its astrological associations, and folklore all become part of the overall formula.

Following is an abbreviated listing of some stones and their uses in healing (both emotional and physical). Those who use crystals recommend that you either hold or carry the token regularly for best results. Some healers also scan the aura with a crystal rather like vacuuming a rug, allowing the stone to collect negativity and interact positively with the energy field. In either case, the crystal should be cleansed and recharged (see "Crystal Treatment," page 127) after each use so no negative energy accidentally flows into the next healing.

Please note that this list includes planetary associations. These can be important for other, less obvious, healing efforts. For example, if someone is feeling tired, healers can potentially use any stone associated with Mars. This planet promotes change, fire, and energy. Similarly, those wishing to improve their ability to give and receive love might choose a crystal aligned with Venus.

Also notice the shapes and sizes of stones when considering their alternative applications. A stone shaped like a heart might help ease an overwhelming feeling of loneliness or loss. One shaped like procreative organs may improve virility under the right circumstances.[4] Nature provides many subtle clues to her workings through color and contour. Combined with your own insight, these often make potent tools, not only for healing, but for many other metaphysical activities.

At the turn of the century, Edgar Cayce suggested that gems may not affect everyone the same way. In effect, Cayce believed that a crystal had to have the right attunement to work physically and spiritually for an individual. This is a very holistic outlook, and one well worth pondering in your own efforts toward crystal healing.

The Crystals

While there are rare gems used in healing, I have limited this list to stones that are more readily obtainable for most people. Additionally, ancient and modern texts sometimes disagree on astrological correspondence. When this happens, both associations are given.

Agate: The immune system; teamwork and harmony (Lunar, Venus, or Mars). In the *Natural History of Precious Stones* (London, 1865), agates are celebrated for their ability to encourage love and a happy home.

Amethyst: Clarity of thought especially on spiritual matters; clearing cold and respiratory complaints (Mercury, Mars,

---

[4]Duffield Osborne, *Engraved Stones* (New York: 1912), p. 138.

or Jupiter). Camilli Leonardi in the *Speculum Lapidum* (1502) stated the belief that amethyst could cure drunkenness, control evil thoughts, and improve intelligence.

Aquamarine: Tension-related difficulties, peace; kidney trouble, right-brain thinking (Venus or Mars). Some historians believe that the stones worn by the high priest of the Second Temple (Exodus 28:15–30, breastplate description) were aquamarines.

Blue topaz: Positive self-images, clarity of ideas, easing tension; the thyroid (Uranus, Saturn, or Mars). St. Hildegard (see earlier this chapter) recommended topaz for vision problems.

Carnelian: Adrenal glands, dietary disorders, lethargy; (Mars, Jupiter, or Venus). In the Far East, Carnelian was used to avert envy. During the Middle Ages, its reddish hue made it a recommended stone for blood ailments.

Coral: Digestive and bladder difficulties; general protective amulet, especially for children and animals (Pluto, Moon, or Mars, if red).

Copper: Circulatory problems; ability to integrate energy or ideas (Sun).

Fire opal: Passion, both physical and intellectual (Pluto, Sun, or Mercury). Albertus Magnus considered the opal to be a stone of honor, able to cure eye disease.[5]

Garnet: Occult studies, karma; memory (Pluto or Sun). Some ancient drinking vessels were made from purplish

---

[5]Lewis Spence, *Encyclopedia of Occultism* (New York: Fireside/Simon and Schuster, 1989), pp. 115–117.

Indian garnet so the beverage within could appear like wine, but in fact be harmless juice!

Gold: While a metal, gold and silver are used as part of the crystal healing process. Gold emphasizes the masculine nature; strength, logic, cleansing fires (Sun).

Jade: The knees, improving relationships and personal joy (Saturn). Native Americans used jade to treat kidney problems. In Guiana, Sir Walter Raleigh recounts the native use of jade for stones. Galen in 130 A.D. wrote, "This is true of the green Jasper, that is to say, this stone aids the stomach and navel by contact."

Lapis: Bravery, averting negative energy; balancing physical energies (Uranus or Venus). The Ebers Papyrus of Egyptian origins encourages the use of lapis as an eye wash.

Malachite: Tooth and mouth problems, improving patience (Saturn). During the Middle Ages, malachite was carried as an amulet to protect one from falling—an especially potent token for horsemen.

Onyx: Assembling research or data; ankles and feet (Moon).

Pearl: Stomach difficulties; forgiveness of self and others (Moon, Venus, or Mercury). Powdered pearl in a wine base was sometimes prescribed as an "all purpose" curative.

Quartz (clear): General all purpose stone, especially good for transmitting energy and improving your "signals" (Sun). John Dee, astrologer to Queen Elizabeth in the 1550s, used a quartz in his healing techniques.

Rose quartz: Heart problems, blood pressure; friendship and developing grace (Mars).

Silver: Nurturing, intuitive (Lunar).

Sugilite: Calming automatic responses/actions; fear (Pluto).

Tiger's eye: Headaches, migraines; focus (Jupiter).

Topaz: Hormone imbalances; renewed optimism and hope (Jupiter). A Roman physician (Arnobio), during the 1600s, recommended topaz for the plague.

Turquoise: Truthful words, sagacity, inventiveness (Uranus, Venus, or Mercury). If one wears turquoise and it begins to fade, this indicates poor health.

Watermelon tourmaline: Originally imported from Sri Lanka around 1700, this version is applied to bring balance into the triune nature, emphasizing Earth healing as part of physical healing.

CRYSTAL THERAPY by Colleen M. Rose CCT[6]

The question people ask me most about crystal therapy is what scientific basis exists for it. Beyond the historical criteria, we do have factual information that acts as a foundation. Crystals are pyroelectric, meaning they literally become electrified or polarized by temperature changes. They are also piezoelectric, meaning they generate voltage under pressure. Beyond these two important characteristics, crystals have surrounding electromagnetic fields and a frequency to which they vibrate. Because of all these attributes, crystals are

---

[6]Used by permission. Affectionately known to those she has helped as the "boo-boo witch," Colleen is a Certified Crystal Therapist and lecturer. For more information on her work write: Colleen Rose, 311 Liberty St., Long Beach, NJ 07740.

widely used in modern science and technology in everything from shortwave radios and lasers to computer chips, watches, ultrasound equipment, condensers, oscillators, and transducers.

The interaction of the crystals on human physicality is understandable when you examine the makeup of our bodies. Human bodies are basically salt and water, salt being a type of crystal. In crystal therapy, one actually affects the liquid crystals of the body through the solid ones formed by Earth. Second, the human body also has an electromagnetic field similar to that of crystals, and it vibrates with specific frequencies as crystals do.

When people are physically, spiritually, or emotionally unbalanced, the electromagnetic field is affected; it does not maintain its normal "curve." This can produce a physical response, namely disease. By applying a crystal with the appropriate electromagnetic field and vibrational frequency, you can move the misaligned arc of energy back into the correct position. This reminds the body's field of how its supposed to run, helping bring things back onto a normal keel.

This is a simple clarification of what crystal therapy is all about. I strongly suggest anyone interested in this field look closely at certification. A full course of study is suggested, including basic geology, chemistry as it applies to crystals, the chakra system, meridians, basic anatomy and physiology, and perhaps even electromagnetic fields as they apply to the human body.

Knowing what a crystal does physically, emotionally, intellectually, and spiritually is simply not enough. You need to know the systems of energy with which you are working to be a responsible, effective healer.

CRYSTAL TREATMENT

When you think of a surgeon's tools, the word sterilized immediately comes to mind. Those working with metaphysical healing need to be no less careful with their own tools. Crystals have the innate ability to collect energy with or without being used. Therefore, cleaning these items before and after each use is paramount to effective, responsible service.

Each person has a different approach to purification. Some place their crystals in a solution of salt water or water with lemon juice for a certain period of time, both salt and lemon being known for their cleansing qualities. The Native American approach is to move the tool through sage smoke, allowing the clouds to carry negativity away. A contemporary pagan might set the stone in the light of the Sun or Moon (or both). Visualizations with white-light energy are also common.

All of these techniques are valid and useful alone, or in combination. They are also effective if you choose to charge your stone with a specific type of energy before working. For example, first douse the crystal in salt water to remove any latent energy, then leave it in the light of a full Moon to improve intuitive, empathic awareness.

Also, when you finish working with a crystal, have a special spot in which to house it away from handling by pets, children, or curious houseguests. I have seen people use everything from ornately carved boxes and satin pouches to fish tanks—the latter being used specifically for water-related stones. Exactly where you choose to tuck your healing stones is a personal choice, but let it reflect the purpose of that crystal in some manner and your own vision.

CRYSTAL MEDITATIONS

Crystals are as unique and multifaceted as people in their own lovely way. Just as you would never expect two rose bushes to grow in exactly the same way, the way crystals develop will change their character, basic matrix, and eventual use in a spiritual setting. Additionally, each crystal has a slightly different message for its user/owner, depending on the need and the situation at hand. Meditation is one key that helps decipher that message.

Begin by choosing one crystal with which to work regularly for a month. You may not need that long, but commit yourself to working with that stone for a full 30-day period. Look at it, hold and feel it daily, see each side and facet in different lighting conditions. Get to know this object with the same tenacity that you might develop a friendship. After all, a familiar tool employed by skilled hands is a friend.

During meditation, lie down and hold the crystal near your navel or place it on your third eye. Speak the name or color of the crystal aloud steadily and repetitively until the room resonates with that energy. When the energy reaches a noticeable level, roll carefully to one side and make notes of what you're feeling. Free-flow writing works very well here; don't try to be overly picky about penmanship or grammar. Repeat this exercise daily, at the same time if possible.

Carry the stone with you until the month is over. Make notes of any changes you perceive in personal behavior or health. Reading these notes, combined with those of your meditations, should provide a pretty strong indication of how this particular crystal should be used for yourself or others.

PLACEMENT OF CRYSTALS

Beyond the type, shape, and color of crystal chosen, various areas on the body are more conducive to specific types of healing than others. Frequently, healers associate these regions with the chakras, or energy centers of the human body. Here is a brief list of those correspondences for your reference.

Crown: Faith, trust, belief; total physical balance.

Third eye: Imagination, creativity, metaphysical insight; associated with the planet Mars, sign of Aries; memory.

Temple: Will; headaches.

Ear: Understanding, discernment; immune system.

Throat: Power, energy, zeal and truthfulness; associated with the planet Venus, sign of Taurus; lungs, respiratory ailments, thyroid.

Solar plexus: Love; associated with Leo and the Sun; addictions.

Stomach: Personal judgment and perspective; associated with the Moon and Cancer; energy and diet.

Lower abdomen: Order, organization; digestion.

Mid-lower back: Strength; associated with Libra and Venus; kidneys.

Upper thigh: Eradicating negative habits or poisons; associated with Pluto and Scorpio; genitals.

Lower thigh: Life energy, vigor; associated with Sagittarius and Jupiter.

Knee: Associated with Capricorn and Saturn; bone and joint problems.

Ankle: Associated with Aquarius and Uranus; circulation.

Bottom of the foot: Associated with Pisces and Neptune; balance and foundations.

BEYOND THE HUMAN EQUATION

Since we will be studying Earth healing later in this book, I want to touch briefly here on the nonhuman uses for crystals too. What about ailing plants and animals? Since they are alive, they also have auric fields that crystals can affect. So, go ahead! Add a specially blessed and charged crystal to your gardens, plant pots, pet beds, and collars. While there is nothing that proves effectiveness 100 percent, the effort certainly can't hurt! In fact, many gardeners I know swear by quartz crystals to improve their yield.

Taking this idea even a little further, what about carrying crystals in your car, or placing them near the TV and around other electrical items? Who knows, just maybe there will be a crystal-healing guidebook for gadgets in the future!

SOURCES FOR CRYSTALS

In shopping for crystals, price does not always insure quality or effectiveness. While in Hindu beliefs, a crystal's clarity improves potency, this also makes a stone terribly expensive. Being in the ministry does not mean being married to poverty in order to obtain tools, so let common sense and your inner voice prevail.

Lightly scan stones you see for their energy. When one jumps off the shelf and into your hands (metaphorically), you can be fairly certain it's "right" for your work. Some of these selections you will keep and reuse; others will be gifts for specific individuals who need them. In both cases, your heart is the best guide in the world for choosing. The Earth has made each crystal and, rather like modern cereal boxes, each one has a surprise inside that you can discover. Just stay aware, open, and sensitive. Here are some good places to look for inexpensively priced stones:

Lapidary shops;
Jewelry stores (faceted stones usually);
Rock shops or gem/mineral societies;
Gem/mineral shows;
College mineralogy professors;
New Age shops;
Science shops (children's nature stores).

7

Divination, Channeling, and Mediumship

Thine was the prophet's vision
—Henry Wadsworth Longfellow

FORTY THOUSAND YEARS AGO, HEALER-PRIESTS
served human tribes in northern Asia. Denoted by the term
"shaman," these people used metaphysical methods to effect cures in their village. One of these methods was trance
healing.

Ancients believed that all illness emanates from the
spirit realm; e.g. wellness directly reflects a positive relationship with the gods. Thus, it was necessary for the shaman to
travel the spirit world to discover restoratives or plead for
aid. In trance healing, the shaman entered an altered state
and mediated between the spirits and the patient, then returned with an appropriate prescription. In other words,
shamans became channels for divine missives.

The term "shaman" originated in the Tunquso-
Manchurian language where *saman* translates roughly into
"one who knows." This connotation remains. Contemporary healer-priests continue a legacy started by some of our
earliest progenitors by allowing themselves to become conduits for Spirit (in any number of forms).

The gifts of channeling, mediumship, and divination pertain mostly to emotional care-givers or to guide-

visionaries. People with these abilities usually serve the emotional and spiritual well-being of their patients versus obtaining actual physical results. However, divination and mediumship may be used to obtain curative information, the most notable practitioner of this method being Edgar Cayce.[1]

Edgar Cayce learned how to place himself into a trance and perform health readings. At first, he did this only for friends. It was not until Cayce cured his own year-long bout of laryngitis, with the help of a hypnotist to guide his trance, that he became a public advocate of psychic phenomena. For the next forty years, he devoted his life to "seeing the body" and making recommendations for healing from this altered state.

Cayce was rare in his devotion to this art, and the way his gift developed was unusual. Nonetheless, I believe that anyone can learn to be an effective medium or diviner with practice and a willingness to set aside his or her own opinions on any matter. It may take time, but we all have access to the higher self, or the collective unconscious of Jung's writings. From this pool of awareness, we can gather in the draught of wellness for those needing aid and a fresh perspective.

For the purpose of this chapter, we will examine channeling, mediumship, and divination in terms of counseling and information retrieval. In the case of the former, psychics use their talents to provide their patients with guidance and advice on any number of emotional or spiritual

---

[1]Edgar Cayce lived during the Victorian era and was called the "sleeping prophet" by his contemporaries. This title reflected his use of trance states to retrieve information on physical conditions and cures for his patients. For his efforts, Cayce never required payment, but suggested a $20 donation. These donations eventually allowed him to establish the ARE (Association for Research and Enlightenment), which continues psychic studies and Cayce's teachings today in Virginia Beach, VA.

matters. For the latter, they seek spiritual insight into the cause of dis-ease (any type), and possible treatments.

In either case, tremendous caution is necessary. Divine missives are not a consistent, reliable source of medical recommendations, no matter our faith in the matter. Further, some regions still have laws regulating "soothsaying" and various forms of divination.[2] Therefore, always advise your clients to keep up with their personal physician's or psychiatrist's orders.

It is also prudent to portray your services in terms of what you believe they can offer, not as 100 percent medically sound. This may seem to surrender the power of your gift to verbal nitpicking, but you can help no one from a jail cell.

CHANNELING AND MEDIUMSHIP

In ancient days, the channel or medium was known by many names and served many functions. At the Greek oracle of Delphi, the Pythia provided divine missives after becoming possessed by Apollo. In Tibet, the state oracle at Nechung is an important aspect of their history in that monks consult the indwelling spirit to find incarnations of the Dalai Lama.[3]

The Babylonian and Hittite civilizations had mediums who became royal counselors. The Japanese consulted village oracles *(takusen matsuri)* annually for information on the rice crop. In all cases, however, the answers gained through the medium's trance state were credited to the gods or goddesses of that culture.

---

[2]Call your town, city, or county office for details. Each region varies. Some areas only prohibit fortune telling without an appropriate business license, while other areas impose fines for any fortune-telling activities.
[3]Michael Loewe and Carmen Blacker, eds., *Oracles and Divination* (Boston: Shambhala, 1981), p. 33.

People believed that a divine being was coaxed through offerings, prayers, and the trance state into temporarily leaving his or her resting place. This being then borrowed the medium's body to answer questions about critical situations for an individual or entire community. This is an important change to note in our studies. You will find very few mediums or channels in modern society who credit their spirit-voice to a specific god or goddess.

In terms of health, the early channels/mediums typically prescribed amuletic cures. From a practical standpoint, this is understandable. Amulets did not directly harm the patient. Conversely a misprescribed curative (like an herbal potion) could result in both the patient's and prophet's death. Amulets also provided hope, which frequently gave the patient temporary relief, thereby proving the oracle's success. If the treatment later failed, it was explained as fate, or lack of faith—certainly not something the oracle could overcome!

Nonetheless, channels and mediums were important to the lives of our ancestors. While rumor and cunning ploys can account for the popularity of some figures, I believe a number of individuals were quite "in tune" with greater forces. Asklepieion of Memphis, for example, was a world-renowned center for oracular healing. People would travel there from miles around praying for a miracle. A goodly number must have found one, or the center's fame would not have spread.

Before examining the modern channel and medium, I feel it important to alleviate some general misconceptions about these arts. In *Webster's New World Dictionary*, one of the definitions for the term channel is: "a frequency band within which a radio or television station must keep its signal." In terms of metaphysics, this means channelers attune their spirits to precise alternate frequencies so they can receive messages (or, potentially, transmit them).

Exactly to what these frequencies equate differs according to your school of thought. Some say this process opens the crown chakra to receive telepathic insights or wisdom from the higher self (see Part II, chapter 3, "Auric Cleansing and Balancing"). Others believe contact takes place between themselves and spirits of various natures. In either case, the information gathered comes from a supernatural source, beyond conventional perceptions.

According to Zolar, "everything is mediumistic, and every atom is a medium for the expression of spiritual force."[4] Fully evolved mediums, therefore, adjust every cell of their bodies temporarily to the task of changing their spiritual frequency. They then collect information and broadcast signals from that frequency like an inter-dimensional telephone line. In other words, they "tap into" specific thought-forms on the astral plane, then communicate those ideas.

In some instances (but not all), this results in mediumship. Mediums in deep trance states act like a party line where one or more voices from Spirit may switch in. Conversely, trans-channeling does not require "possession" by the spirit to be effective. Instead, psychics reach meditative states, listen to the missive from Spirit, then convey that message themselves. I have used this technique successfully to write particularly difficult portions of a book. The only difference is in having fingers and typewriter keys transmit the message instead of my mouth!

To me, trans-channeling offers many improvements over traditional mediumship. In the case of the latter, accountability can be lost. After all, how do you track down a disincarnate spirit to confront them about misinformation?

On the other hand, the trans-channel chooses to relay a message in whole or in part. If personal predispositions or opinions get mixed in, the responsibility falls directly in the channeler's lap, where it belongs. To balance this statement, there are numerous reliable mediums who only work

---

[4]Zolar; *Encyclopedia of Ancient and Forbidden Knowledge* (New York: Fireside/Simon and Schuster, 1989), p. 142.

with specific entities that they trust from repeated experience. The key here is in finding an individual with a solid reputation.

CHANNELING by Colleen M. Rose CCT[5]

I have been doing channeling since 1981. In that time, I have seen the energies that work through me help individuals produce astounding changes in their lives. Even more significant to me, however, were the changes experienced in my own life thanks to these channeled energies.

While I am not versed in physics, toe fungus, or sacred geometry, channeling opens those worlds. Yet, beyond this I find one piece of channeled information most intriguing as to why there are so many channels appearing today. The answer was: We are not here to attune humankind's ears to one voice, or any one energy. We are here and we speak to attune humankind to Truth. To remind your ears of what Truth sounds like, feels like, smells like, tastes like, looks like and vibrates like. There is coming a time when you will all need the knowledge of the being called Truth.

The implication of all five senses plus one being present within one greater sense—Truth—was enough in itself. But realizing that Truth, in a greater sense, has a kind of life essence, took me back. It still does. This kind of awareness is what channeling offers to us, and in the process tends to keep egos in check.

Drawbacks

No matter which title you go by, if channeling or mediumship is your choice of healing art, be prepared for some difficult situations. Many people seeking a channeler are hungry for "supernatural" experiences. This, in itself, is not

[5]Used by permission.

a bad thing. However, there is a danger in allowing a dependency to develop. I call this "guru awe," where people rely on psychic information as their only guidance instead of trusting their heart and inner voice.

In extreme cases, individuals won't even leave the house without reading their horoscope and checking with their psychic first. They spend thousands of dollars seeking readers to put bandages on all of life's bumps and bruises. This actually hinders real personal growth. So, when you see someone coming to you too frequently, find a gentle way to encourage a little soul searching. Remember, a healer's ultimate job is to teach people to heal themselves.

The second disadvantage to channeling and mediumship is a substantial energy drain for the healer after every session. For some reason, the physical and psychic exertion in this technique seems more pronounced. This is why many mediums and channels limit the number of sittings they have in one day, and schedule them carefully to allow recuperative time.

Also, mediums and channels, by their very nature, are more open to spiritual messages than most people. This means they are likely to receive communications for their patients outside of normally scheduled sessions. Unfortunately, this can become very disruptive to their privacy and concentration. Here's one true story. The names have been fictionalized upon request.

The Office Visit

"Sue" was at the office in the middle of an important project when a friend's spirit guide showed up. She was worried by the guide's sudden appearance. So, "Sue" excused herself immediately and called her friend, "Bob," to make sure he was all right.

When she discovered her friend was home, casually watching TV, it was a relief, but one that produced a fount of righteous anger. "Sue" proceeded to rather tactlessly blast "Bob" for his lack

of spiritual listening skills. She then told those entities, in no un-
certain terms, not to appear at the office again unless it was a mat-
ter of life and death.

This story dramatically illustrates one of the hardest lessons for most channels and mediums to learn: how to say "no" to Spirit when necessary.

Another difficulty facing those who become effective mediums is the spirit of disbelief and what I call the "side-show effect." In the former, someone brings you a referral who obviously has little faith in what you're about to do. In this case, you need to consider if it's truly worth the time and energy to try. Some people's opinions can be dramatically transformed by one positive experience; others' cannot. It will be up to your sensitivities to decide what's best here.

In the second scenario, someone has come to you without a real need; they want to either poke fun at the "New Age geek" or just experience something different. Under these circumstances, I see no reason to perform like a trained dog. There is every reason to honor your abilities by not allowing them to be randomly abused.

A fourth problem with channeling and mediumship is the source of information. The majority of entities contacted during these moments are disincarnate spirits who have to return to the Earth plane. This means that the soul is still subject to all human flaws. Their after-life missives and health advice may prove no more helpful than a casual conversation with them did when they were alive. After all, not every spirit has been a physician in a past incarnation!

This sometimes leaves the channel seeking devic[6] or master-teacher spirits for consultation, who tend to be

---

[6]Devas are powerful nature spirits who are very old and exist as part of Earth's sacred sphere. Their insights can be quite startling, since they can observe the human state from the outside.

much more trustworthy. Alternatively, they must hone their intuitive senses to know which spirits are offering *real* aid, by no means an easy task. These circumstances encourage mediums and channels to set up protected spaces for themselves that restrain negative influences (see "The Process" later this chapter).

Advantages

The advantages to channeling are truly a marvel to behold. For a moment, you move into another realm of awareness, a psychic pool,[7] from which insights may be collected. Here, the self steps aside to discern matters of import hidden from our physical awareness. These glimpses may not always make sense or seem important to the channel, but they can prove amazingly essential to a client in distress. The following anecdote gives one example.

Melinda's Story[8]

A young woman went to a channeler, feeling unhappy and depressed without an apparent reason. Her energy and zeal had waned steadily over the past few months until she found it difficult to get out of bed. Nothing inspired her; nothing seemed to really matter.

The channeler was baffled, knowing Melinda to be a healthy, intelligent woman. She began to meditate and open herself to Spirit's impressions, which often came in the form of a picture or texture. In this instance, her spirit guide provided an odd clue, the feeling of rich soil between her fingers, and a soaring emotion of joy

---

[7]C. G. Jung called this the collective unconscious, where all the learning and knowledge of the ages can potentially be tapped.
[8]The following three stories are true. The actual names of the clients and psychic readers were withheld by request.

afterward. At this point, the channeler wondered if she'd misinterpreted the impression, as it made no sense. Nothing else came through, so she reiterated the message, adding that she wasn't totally sure of its accuracy.

By this time Melinda was crying. Tears of happiness flowed freely from her, leaving the channeler even more confused than before! Then, Melinda explained that some time ago she'd considered moving to the country and starting her own farm. She was unhappy at work and with living in the city. Melinda loved working with the land, but felt a farm was only an impractical pipe dream. Spirit basically told her that satisfaction and fulfillment would be found in that dream and to follow it.

Melinda's entire demeanor changed within those few moments. The same woman who dragged herself into the room earlier now stood tall and confident, smiling broadly. Eight months later, Melinda was living happily on her farm, never once regretting her decision.

This story potently displays how channels and mediums relay information that can plant the seeds for new ideas and projects, or water those already present. Here the channel goes to Spirit and returns with practical, positive input. Channels can also provide that all-important message of hope, giving people renewed determination to keep trying.

A second advantage of channeling and mediumship is a unique understanding of the world beyond the grave. I think one of the most common areas of anxiety for many people is what happens to them after they die. For the medium and channel, the answer is firm; we move onward.

The ability to speak with the dead has several applications. First, when mediums and channels become the voices for deceased loved ones, they provide emotional healing to the living through relief and hope. Second, mediums sense spiritual imbalances affecting homes or whole areas. They then listen to the spirits there, collect information, and discuss what actions they believe will cure that astral "sickness." The following story demonstrates how.

Bump in the Night

We got a call one day, saying a friend's home seem plagued with slamming doors and terrible drafts coming from nowhere. The caller asked if Taka and I would consider taking a look-see. They knew both Taka and I had experience with a few ghosts before, and his shamanistic training might be necessary.

So we went out there, with sage incense and a few protective amulets, not really expecting to find anything. While other people checked out the cellar, I remained in the kitchen with my daughter. As I stood at the bottom of a staircase, a rush of cold air poured downward. A spirit-child stood at my feet. He told me his name was Michael.

I called Taka, but something had caught his attention elsewhere. While I waited, the scene of Michael falling down the stairs and breaking his neck became painfully clear to me. Michael was not an angry spirit, but he desperately wanted his Mommy and his toys. I could not sense his mother anywhere and, as for the toys . . . well I hoped we could find something appropriate.

By this time Taka had returned, stating that a tree in the back yard had to be taken out completely. Someone had been hung there during the Civil War and the taint of anger was poisoning the ground. Apparently Michael's uncle had hanged a trespasser the same day he'd arrived with a rocking horse for the boy—the same day that Michael died. The power of this information was so overwhelming that the people with us who did not believe in ghosts could actually feel the changes in the house as they occurred.

As we discussed our feelings and experiences, we noticed that the owners of the house had a rocking horse in the living room. We moved this immediately to the kitchen where the rush of cold air was felt again afterward. Michael was playing happily. The spirit of his uncle was less restless now too, seeing joy come from the gift that had originally caused Michael to fall down the stairs in excitement.

Upon further inspection we discovered one more spirit abiding upstairs. This was the child's grandmother, who just wanted some flowers to enjoy. This was her home, and she would not leave it . . . but flowers would make her happy. We found a small bundle of wild blossoms on the dining room table and moved them accordingly. Looking to the kitchen, we could still sense Michael playing there and his uncle looking on protectively. Once the tree was taken out of the yard, we believed this house and the surrounding land would be whole again.

By the time we left, the entire area was showing signs of renewed vitality. The smell of pine filled the air and the gloom that had pierced every corner earlier seemed all but gone. Someone knew these people's stories now—so the spirits could rest. The family living in that house has had no problems since.

Another advantage to channeling and mediumship is more personal in nature. Because of the realm in which this gift operates, channels are more regularly in touch with their own higher selves and guides. In traveling astral paths, they glean many insights that can aid their own growth.

Many times channelers express wonder at the messages they've conveyed. Within those communiqués, specific needs in their own lives and hearts can also be met. In this manner, Spirit serves metaphysical meals to two tables at once, leaving both parties filled and refreshed.

DIVINATION

Divination is defined as trying to determine the unknown through a specific medium. Looking more closely at this term we see two distinct roots, both of which explain its meaning in metaphysical terms: "divine" comes from the Latin word *(divus)* for a god, or something from god;

"-ation" means the act of, or the condition of being. In other words, diviners strive to perform a function similar to that of channelers and mediums in that they become one with divine energy during a reading.

From earliest history, the most prevalent types of divination were those derived from omens and signs. Since animistic faiths believed the wind, storms, animals, and other living objects had spirits, it was natural to look to these powers for helpful harbingers. Individuals who became adept at reading these signs became priests, who then tried to use their abilities to extend life and improve its quality.

Some ancient divination methods for health or prognosis include:

The Greeks and Romans using the sound of wind through oak leaves as an oracle.

The patterns made by cracking bones and shells was popular in China from 1400–1100 B.C. Sometimes known as scapulimancy or plastromancy, patterns moving upward or to the right portended a better chance of recovery for the patient.

In Tibet, people traveled for hundreds of miles to visit an adept *mopa*, or diviner, who was usually an elderly female. The *mopa* used any number of popular tools to obtain an answer, including arrows, dice, butter lamps, the movement of birds, mirrors, and rosary-type beads.

Placing vervain against the forehead of a patient, and asking, "How do you fare?" This herb allows the patient to answer if he or she will live or die.

In Greece, finding various colored feathers meant different things. Brown ones, especially if found on the right, meant improved health or continued good health. Black ones portended death, especially if found on the left.

Traveling to a Shinto or Buddhist shrine in 15th-century Japan to receive a symbolic dream. Some might consider this method closer to channeling, but since it is not a *conscious* reception on the sleeper's part, I've included it here.

Across the centuries, this idea did not fade, it simply transformed slightly. Animism was less prevalent, but the abiding belief in spiritual causes for disease continued. People sought out gifted individuals with prophetic sight for curatives, no matter how unusual the tools or procedures. Some diviners opted for tarot cards or runes. Others chose crystal balls, augury, or astrology. Still others used dust, the sound of burning herbs, and observations of chickens to make determinations.

The instances of such approaches have declined drastically in modern history, partially due to improved diagnostic procedures within medicine. However, remote areas where both money and medicine are scarce demonstrate a greater frequency of these techniques being used. In China, as recently as 100 years ago, healers utilized medicine sticks to ascertain disease and treatment. For this, the patient selected one of eighteen sticks, each with its own emblem. The sufferer's choice of stick and emblem portended the prognosis.

In another example, the shamans of Nepal still use a brass plate dotted with rice while reciting special mantras. They slowly sort the rice using sacred sounds to guide them in divining the pattern for wellness in their patients. Or, you might find a dowser in England or the United States using rods to locate areas of disease. No matter the approach, the goal is the same; to ascertain the problem and offer ideas for a potential cure.

Different forms of divination provide vastly different amounts of information. Healers must therefore limit their aid to what is feasible considering their tools. Dowsing may reveal much about the source of a problem, but gives us few clues about treatment. Scrying, on the other hand, can furnish symbolic indicators for both parts of the equation.

Drawbacks

Divination has definite limitations. Your tools, being sensitive to energy, sometimes provide wonderful readings that prove totally inaccurate. Alternatively, the actions of the querent can drastically alter the web of fate at any time after the reading. Following is one example where a little of both occurred.

Michael's Reading

Michael was very lonely and wondering if he would ever find someone with whom to share his life. His emotional health was terrible, he lacked confidence and drive, and was rapidly losing hope. So, he asked a friend to read his cards.

The reading indicated that a dark-haired woman would be entering his life within eighteen months. While the psychic was hesitant to promise anything, the cards showed that a long-term commitment was extremely likely. Michael was both relieved and excited. His attitude over the ensuing months improved greatly.

After eighteen months, no woman had surfaced. Michael returned to his reader to inquire further. The diviner pulled another card that portended a waiting period. It was just too soon. Finally, six months later, a woman fitting the original description appeared. She was a loving, giving person who would happily have nurtured Michael through his insecurities. But Michael felt she was not his physical "ideal," so he broke things off within weeks, even though the relationship worked marvelously.

It took months for both individuals to recover emotionally from this situation. Michael suffered from guilt pangs and the woman felt used. Years later, these people, while cordial to each other in public, still have trouble being in the same room together.

So what exactly happened here? First, Michael's hopeful anticipation poured over into the runes and "pushed up" the time frame so it was inaccurate. Second, Michael did not realize that, when the universe answers our needs, it is not necessarily in an idyllic form. In this case, the reading was basically accurate. Michael was given a potential soulmate. Unfortunately, his surprising reaction to this answer completely changed the outcome from what had been was predicted. That's the way free will works.

Because of these kinds of limitations, it is a good idea to advise your clients of potential variances. Everything they do from the moment of the reading forward can, and does, change the future. Matters of health are even more sensitive to our actions (or lack thereof). Approaching your reading in this manner also encourages your patients to remain active participants in their own well-being instead of just blindly accepting advice.

Other limitations to divinatory arts include the querent's doubts and lack of understanding about why and how specific symbolic tools work. Those unfamiliar with the tarot may find your reading very interesting, but also very confusing. To them, the Major Arcana might just as well be a group of musicians!

If your patients have no emotional or cognitive connection to your divination system, a little more diligence and explanation may be required. Educate your patients about the system you use and why. Eventually they may learn enough from your example to do brief readings for themselves. Alternatively, learn several systems and allow them to choose one with which they personally relate.

Advantages

The nicest thing about divination is that it can take place nearly anywhere with little fuss. Most divination tools are not cumbersome and are rather nonthreatening in their appearance. So, unlike mediumship, which is very awkward in public places, divination can be enacted anywhere that you feel comfortable. This allows diviners to be more spontaneous. They can meet people's needs when they arise, instead of having to wait for a more appropriate time or place.

Additionally, divination tools can be put neatly away between readings. Unlike mediums, who sometimes feel overwhelmed by their sensitivity to missives from the astral realm, diviners can use the storage procedure to "turn off" their gifts temporarily. Since the tool acts as a mental and spiritual prompt, when the tool "rests," so can they.

CHANNELING AND DIVINATION— THE PROCESS

For channeling and mediumship, the individual is the vehicle or tool for the reading. In divination, an object or specific instrument is used for gathering information, while the "reader" observes and interprets that information. Despite these basic differences, the procedures for channeling and divination have striking similarities.

Both healers take time to get prepared through any one of the empowering activities detailed in Part I, chapter 2. Some healers also believe setting up a protective field of energy is important at this point. This sphere keeps out unwanted influence and holds in the healing energy so none is wasted. Exactly what approach each healer uses to create this sacred space varies, although the approach chosen usually mirrors religious patterns, like prayer or invocations.

Next, it is helpful for patients to have specific questions. If they experience repeated knee problems, for example, their question would be: "Why do I have knee problems and how do I correct them?" This query may be voiced aloud or kept private. There are advantages to both approaches.

In divination, sometimes the symbols that appear in a reading make little sense without a context. On the other hand, knowing a question can cause a reader to communicate their own subconscious ideas on the topic instead of those from Spirit.

Channelers are not immune to this "catch-22." Since Spirit communicates to (or through) them, personal opinion can become an issue. For this reason, I generally recommend that questions remain unvoiced until after the session. If for some reason the communiqué is unclear, articulate the question during the reading to help clarify what Spirit is saying.

The third step is actually seeking out, or opening yourself to, the response. In all instances, it is essential that the diviner and channeler remain in control. I have heard horror stories from friends about Ouija boards that conveyed terrible, frightening messages. This should never have occurred.

The minute an entity or reading becomes threatening, or so negative that it creates dread and worry, stop the effort immediately. Whatever energies were contacted in this situation obviously have their own agenda, and do not have the best interests of your patient in mind (see "Drawbacks" earlier in this chapter). When this occurs, if you have not created a protected sphere, do so before trying again. If you did set up a safe zone, try reinforcing it or changing your location.

Changing your location can also help when you find your efforts repeatedly failing for no apparent reason. Some regions of a home, or land, are simply not conducive to spiritual workings of any kind. Perhaps there is too much negativity in this place, a natural energy field that causes static, or a "null" energy field that dampens the lines of communications. In all three cases, moving your session elsewhere usually fixes the problem.

If this is not the case, there is a reason for the silence from Spirit—a reason which should be honored. The person you're working with may need some personal reflection or growth before their question can be answered (and accepted). Or the lines of fate may simply be too tangled right now to provide a reasonably certain response.

When an answer from Spirit comes, it is important for channelers, mediums, and diviners to take a cue from caregivers in their approach. Spirit's messages can be very hard pills to swallow and they are intimate in nature. Our words must be gentle, encouraging, and positive to help patients integrate what they're hearing.

Perhaps Spirit indicated that your patient's cold has to do with falsehood in his or her communications with people. These "little white lies" manifest as a cough. This is not the time to turn to your patient and say "Stop lying!" The accusation will immediately put that individual on the defensive and keep the message from being received at all.

A better way of approaching this message might be to say:

> Spirit indicates that sometimes you're inaccurate in the way you communicate with others. You need to examine your words carefully. As your communications become more accurate, the cough will dissipate.

By a little creative rewording, you can convey the same point, but give the patient a goodly amount of "liquid" with which to swallow Spirit's pill! Additionally, no matter what answer Spirit provides, it must be balanced with an appropriate encouragement for the patient to continue with a regular, prescribed course of treatment.

Once diviners or mediums complete their work, a ritual grounding and cleansing often ensues. Grounding helps bring them back to a normal level of awareness. Stretching, eating crunchy foods (like vegetables), having a glass of cool water, and sitting on the ground all help to reestablish foundations.

Cleansing is a way of dissipating any residual energy from the diviners' tools or, in the case of mediums, themselves. This is an important step because it ensures random energy isn't left lingering. It also ensures that the individual or tool is free from any external influences before the next reading.

Physicians wouldn't dream of prescribing the same medication randomly to all their patients. Similarly, specific frequencies of energy (the spiritual prescription) will not help everyone with whom the diviner/medium works. So, the old energy is cleaned out, leaving a purified, ready vessel.

Finally, a discussion period after a reading is beneficial to both patient and psychic. Some channels don't remember specifics about the session because of the energy they're dealing with.[9] Diviners don't always have the chance to take notes on their readings to double-check their accuracy later. Patients may not have been able to absorb the information as quickly as it was presented. Thus, reflective conversation helps everyone.

---

[9]Consider recording your sessions. This way, all participants can review the tape, step-by-step, stopping to ask questions and getting clarification. The tape then becomes a permanent record of your successful readings.

8

Earthly Realms

*All particles . . . can be created from energy and can
vanish into energy. . . . The whole universe appears as
a dynamic web of inseparable energy patterns.*
—Fritjof Capra

MOST PEOPLE WOULD NEVER CONSIDER DUMPING
trash on a neighbor's lawn. Yet that is exactly how we have
treated this planet—like a giant trash heap for our ex-
pended toys. If people had been hired by the gods as con-
scientious caretakers, I suspect they would have been fired
at least 50 years ago for poor performance.

In our "good intentioned" efforts to make our lives
simpler or better, we have stretched the planet's resources
beyond their limits. The drastic side of this picture is
plainly visible in the raping of the rain forest, oil spills,
landfills, and hazardous-waste dumps. The subtler side is
not always as easy to discern.

I went to a friend's house one day recently and noticed
that his lawn was overgrown. I immediately wondered what
might be wrong. When asked, my friend informed me that
he was tired of hurting the Mother. To him, cutting the
lawn was like shaving off your hair once a week with dull
blades!

I found this concept somewhat drastic but intriguing.
For all my good intentions, did I really consider our planet

as an entity? Air cycles closely resemble respiration in humans, but stones as bones, soil as flesh, and grass as hair? Dan's words kept ringing in my mind until I saw the glorious beauty of his perspective. With one small gesture, he had taught me that little things can and do make a difference to our planet. Gaia deserves to be treated with the same respect as any living thing.

For all intents and purposes, people are the "mind" of Gaia—we make the decisions for this planet in the way we choose to live, in the products we buy or use, and in the way we treat each other. Whether or not this is what the gods intended is uncertain, but that is the powerful role we have taken in Earth's life. Now the question remains as to how responsible we're willing to be. The purpose of Earth healers is taking up that responsibility by serving Gaia's ailing body and spirit, and also by retraining her mind—the human race.

Gaia's hands-on healers dedicate their lives to finding solutions to Earth's growing problems, knowing full well that people will never be whole if the Earth is not likewise so. What ecospiritualists try to inspire is a motivational vision of the future wherein we return to an Earth-friendly, Earth-first attitude. Historically speaking, this is often a thankless job, misunderstood by the populace, and misrepresented by politicians. Henry David Thoreau and the Transcendentalists of the 1800s were good examples. Thoreau's contemporaries ridiculed him for wishing to live simply, in harmony with nature. Today *Walden* is a "classic."[1] Nonetheless, we still haven't learned the lesson he tried to teach over 100 years ago!

---

[1] I highly recommend that every New Age seeker read this book. My copy is tattered and dog-eared from over twenty years of reflective reading.

HISTORY OF ECOSPIRITUALITY

Thoreau was by no means the first writer to challenge the human condition. Many early philosophers, artists, visionaries, and country wise people all had one voice on the subject of nature. Actually, physical manifestations of Earth worship and writings about Earth's spirit are plentiful and very insightful.

Megaliths and spiral stone carvings dot the countryside as a nearly timeless tribute to an early reverence toward the Earth Mother and her inherent power. The mythologies of many cultures also reflect this theme. For example, in Zuni, Navajo, and rural European beliefs, souls wait for rebirth underground—in Earth's womb. One cannot help but wonder what soil pollution does to defile those lingering spirits. Similarly, in China and South America, immediately after birth, mothers place their children on the ground to show them their true parentage.

In the third century, a Greek philosopher named Porphyry spoke about trees having souls. A seventh century Celtic hermit named Marban found God among trees and in the company of birds. St. Anthony (A.D. 250–356) felt that nature was God's open book, to be read. Then there is St. Francis of Assisi (1100s), who is basically the patron saint of ecologists.

St. Francis treated all living things as his "brothers and sisters." His loving service and care for all creation through hands-on efforts was unquestionably an example of what Gaia's healers can accomplish. Even on his deathbed he exclaimed in almost New Age fashion: "Be praised, my lord, for all your creatures! In the first place for the blessed Brother sun . . . for our sister, Mother Earth who nourishes and watches us."[2]

---

[2]Julien Green, *God's Fool: The Life and Times of St. Francis of Assisi* (San Francisco: HarperSanFrancisco, 1985), p. 254.

In the 1400s, when the first immigrants traveled to the New World, they found a group of naturalists waiting for them. The Native Americans had a personal relationship with the Earth and tried to live in communion with its spirit. To them, every valley and rock stirred with the memories of their people; the land was holy. Man and nature were permanently joined in the network of life. Around the same time, a European alchemist named Basilius Valentinus taught that the Earth was inhabited by a spirit or soul from which every living thing draws strength.

In the 1600s, a Jesuit named Jean-Pierre deCaussade tried to simplify the Western outlook by explaining that God could be found in every moment. DeCaussade's ideas were mirrored in both the 1700s and 1800s by Alphonsus and Thérèse of Lisieux, respectively. The former reminisced about God in everything from washwater to firelight, while the latter wrote about the "book of nature."[3]

By the 1800s, nearly every writer and artist seemed to catch a bit of the "natural" bug. The spirit of romance and love of nature were plainly evident. One poet, William Cullen Bryant, even went so far as to call the forests "god's first temples."

As late as 1920, central-African medicine men had to be consulted before cutting down a tree. Even once a blessing was given, sacrifices had to be made to the tree spirit in appeasement. Similarly, in Indonesia, little homes filled with gold, miniature clothes, and food are made for tree spirits before a forest is cleared to plant rice. A remarkable

---

[3]Thérèse de Lisieus'original name was Marie-Francois Thérèse Martin. She was a French Carmelite nun, canonized in 1925. Alphonsus lived from 1696–1787. He was a musician, poet, and theologian.

agriculturalist by the name of William Carver also living in the early part of the century, explained gently to his visitors that touching a flower is touching infinity.

Skipping ahead to the 1960s, Cleve Backster began doing research on plants to measure their response to stimuli using a lie detector. Much to his surprise, he found that supplying water brought a reaction similar to relief, and fire caused a reaction something akin to panic. While his results are still somewhat questionable, they led to a number of interesting experiments about the effects of music, sound, and other stimuli on the plant kingdom. The outcome? Plants seem to like soft, happy music versus sad, boring, or harsh tones.

The United Nations created the World Charter for Nature in 1982. This charter offers guidelines for protecting the planet's environment. It states that harmony with nature provides us all with an opportunity to develop our inventiveness. It also reaffirms that every form of life is unique and worthy of respect.

In 1983, the World Council of Churches asked its members to consider the integrity of all creation as a topical discussion. In 1987, Pope John Paul tackled the environmental crisis, stating that human dominion over the Earth was not absolute—that we do not have the freedom to misuse this gift. The people of Texas seem to agree. In 1990, they sentenced a man to nine years in jail for his crime against nature; purposely killing an old oak tree.

In contemporary India, there is a growing group of Hindus called Chipko who put themselves physically between foresters and the trees. These individuals are trying to stop the deforestation of India because they feel so strongly about their kinship with the trees and all life forms. The term Chipko means literally "to embrace"—a very apt description for hands-on healing!

Today, the Scottish people continue to build their roads through the mountains *around* trees out of respectfulness. All of these people, and many more, bear the same message: creation and god are one and the same.

A JOB DESCRIPTION

Earth healers see the planet as analogous to a human body and deserving of being treated with equal dignity. When one part of the whole is hurt, the entire system of living creatures is affected. This interdependence creates a network wherein we drink particles of the same water that fell on Moses.[4] In essence, we engage in a partnership that is inescapable, but generally unacknowledged.

Ecospirituality is a holistic model wherein the human equation for Earth gets adjusted into balance. Ecospirituality is a dynamic, active, educational process that must have idealism, sound values, realistic attitudes, and active intervention to be effective. Simplified living, finding Earth-friendly technology, respecting the Earth's resources, and changing wasteful behaviors all constitute the foundations of what Gaia's healers hope to achieve in the human condition. These people challenge us to think globally, live globally, and love globally every day. They remind us that the Earth is, indeed, our mother.

Gaia's servants are not simply disembodied voices. They are activists with a "hands-on" approach. These people realize that words alone cannot keep Earth's fragile ecosystem intact. For Humpty Dumpty to remain safely on his wall, we have to start actively working together, not just talking about it.

---

[4]Ken Wilber, in *The Holographic Paradigm and Other Paradoxes* (Shambhala, 1988, p. 250), says that "each time we breathe we take in a quadrillion atoms breathed by the rest of the human race within the last two weeks."

The Human Body in the Planet Body[5]

Working with my husband on the Earthen Spirituality Project has allowed me to participate in planetary healing as I would never have imagined possible. For over two decades, Jesse Wolf Hardin has taught and written about the process of reconnection and awareness with Gaia that also helps fulfill personal power. Here, in the mother's womb, he has helped me and others find the most potent, real magic of all.

Gaian healing is founded on the deepest experiencing of the human body as part of the planetary body. Herein, we learn to recognize and consciously embrace our membership in this body. From this perspective, it is clear that the only effective system of personal healing is tapping the energies of Gaia. Crystals garner their energy from the Earth; herbs are informed gifts from the Earth; spiritual midwifery involves Earth-grounding and empowerment; spells work because they are Earthen prayers. Likewise, there can't be any sustainable personal healing without simultaneously treating our larger body: this ailing, sacred Earth.

Mental and physical disease are conditions of planetary or personal imbalance. Every act of healing thus becomes a matter of moving energy in such a way that it restores that balance. One of the long-term obstacles to human health is the untreated cultural imbalance in which we live. You cannot hope to cure an individ-

---

[5]Used by permission. Loba G. Hardin, Earthen Spirituality Project. Loba Hardin is the life partner of Jesse Wolf Hardin, a renowned writer and speaker on ecospirituality. The Earthen Spirituality Project [ESP] is dedicated to Gaian reconnection and Earth-awareness. They offer workshops, lectures, and the opportunity to apprentice in the Gila Mountains. Write them through Llewellyn Publications, Box 64383, St. Paul, MN 55164-0383 for more information. Jesse Hardin's books include: *Full Circle: A Song of Ecology and Earthen Spirituality* (St. Paul, MN: Llewellyn, 1991, 1-800-843-6666); *Totem: Animal Teachers & the ReWilding of Humanity* ($24.00 through ESP); *The Kokopelli Seed* (novel, $24.00, through ESP); *Oikos: Songs for the Living Earth* ($12.00 tape, $16.00 CD, from ESP).

ual without treating other "carriers"—in this case, one's family, community, or the whole planet.

Until recently, councilors have encouraged people to try to "live with" society rather than changing it. Gaian healers advise just the opposite. As part of this planetary being, we have a responsibility to change and treat the whole. When we do, nothing less than miracles result.

MAKING ROOM FOR GOD

Our forefathers regarded nature as the perfect reflection of divine ideas, patterns, and lessons. Even as little as a century ago, this meant honoring the Earth by living in reciprocity. People gave thanks for their food, for the harvest, for rain and sunlight. How often do we remember to give thanks today?

Have we become so busy, and our world so overcrowded, that there seems to be little room left for a grateful heart or for the gods of our forefathers? An important aspect of ecospirituality is that it challenges this entire trend. We need to dive into our collective soul as a race and welcome the sacred back into the world.[6]

Gaia's healers return our attention to the Earth-centered mental framework of our ancestors. Herein, the divine is a transcendent power with which we strive to re-unite in order to discover fulfillment. Since this power is in all things, we cannot separate ourselves from nature, or continue abusing her resources, and hope to find god. In other words, we must make room for god; room where this being may exhibit universal lessons through creation.

---

[6]See C. G. Jung's concept of the collective unconscious, *The Portable Jung* (New York: Viking, 1971), pp. 59ff.

Drawbacks

There are certain cautions that Gaia's healers must bear in mind. Nature has her own sense of checks and balances. In a self-regulated system, any external interference may make matters worse. So sometimes, our efforts to undo the past may not be well placed. This is where ecospiritualists must acquire a keen ear and eye to subtle signals from the natural world to know when to help and when to leave well-enough alone.

The best example I have of this is the annual cycle of whale beachings that occurs in Australia. When environmental rescue workers came to help these creatures back into the seas, the aborigines were horrified. In their beliefs, the whales on the beach were a gift from the gods[7]—the gift of food and many other useful items. When such a creature was discovered, no part of it was ever wasted, and it was received with thankfulness.

I cannot say for certain whose attitude is correct. The rescue workers want to offer the animal life—but what will happen when they return to sea? The aborigines want to offer the animal honor in death. Both outlooks have merit. The question then becomes, what is the greatest good? What does the universe ask of us?

GLOBAL HEALING—THE VISION

Nearly everyone involved in ecospirituality agrees that environmental activism is an important component for global healing. There is a very real correlation between the Earth's condition and the human spiritual state. When we stop exploiting each other, we will likely stop exploiting the Earth—it is really that basic. Nonetheless, this atonement

---

[7] *Undersea Worlds*, The Discovery Channel.

requires a drastic change from our materialistic society into one based on an ideal of love and justice.

Gaia's healers see beyond this societal horizon, or they could never do their job. They envision global healing as a process that includes, but is not limited to:

Affirmation of a divine presence in the universe, our world, and in ourselves;

Seeking out that divinity and actively emulating it so that the beings of this planet become more light-filled;

Fighting against injustice to bring transformation. It is impossible to achieve global healing without some direct intervention.

APPLIED ECOSPIRITUALITY

As with all other forms of healing studied in this text, Gaia's healers each have an approach that suits their ideals, knowledge, and talents. The diversity evidenced in these methods is amazing, yet the congruity in their meaning is even more astounding. Here are some examples:

Feng Shui: Feng Shui comes from China. It is basically an art form that seeks to bring human structures into harmony with their natural surroundings. The people who practice Feng Shui use their understanding of *qi* (the Earth spirit) to respectfully adjust a room or a whole town's placement. The changes they make are purposeful, treating their project and the *qi* as part of a single system. This adjustment improves the quality of life through the ensuing positive flow of *qi*.

Sacred Geometry: Similar in many ways to Feng Shui, sacred geometry studies the natural lines of energy pulsating through the Earth known as Ley lines. The theory behind Ley lines was first proposed in 1921 by a Welshman named Alfred Watkins. After traveling for many years, Watkins concluded that many sacred sites throughout the world were placed along specific directional lines that could be charted. By studying those lines, one could chart Gaia's auric energy.

Sacred geometry has done just that. In the process, it has reawakened people's latent awareness of telluric energy and how it affects us. Sacred geometrists use their knowledge to reconnect Ley lines that have been broken or bent from human endeavors. This helps return energy to Earth, even as unblocking an artery returns blood to a wanting vein, or as Shiatsu and accupressure returns the meridians to an all-connected state (see Part II, chapter 1).

Biodynamic Farming: Foundational to this approach is a belief that not all of Earth's energies are understood or acknowledged. People practicing this art replenish their soil annually by using organic composts so their crops can be healthy. Food grown in this soil is then believed to be more nutritional, better tasting, and spiritually enriching to both body and soul.

Biodynamic farming had its beginnings in the 1920s with Rudolf Steiner, an Austrian scientist. He began by instructing people on the dangers of certain "modern" farming methods, specifically that artificial fertilizers were killing the soil. Steiner was an advocate of using cosmic energy in a beneficial manner.

To this end, he stressed biodynamic soil solutions that were spiritually energized. These preparations were homeopathic in nature, having both real and symbolic importance to the farming process. Not long after his lectures began in 1924, biodynamics became part of the popular culture. During the 1960s, Dan Carlson continued Steiner's studies, adding to them the concepts of harmonics. His approach is now being tested around the world with positive results.

Today, the best remaining evidence we have of this thinking are cooperatives and healthfood stores. More people are turning to untreated foods to keep their bodies free from chemicals. They are also returning to the pharmacy of Earth to cure their ills.

Ritualistic Efforts: Ritual is a means of honoring the sacred. For many people in the New Age community, it offers a way to give something back to the land and channel positive energy for Earth-healing.

Ritualistic approaches vary from person to person, even among those walking similar paths. One person might plant blessed crystals in the ground, then encircle their parcel of land while singing, dancing, or chanting. Another may pour out a specially prepared herbal mixture on a tree they have named "Earth." In both instances, individuals use their actions metaphorically to direct healthy vibrations to the whole planet.

Empowered Visualization: This entails visualizing a whole, united Earth and extending healing energy to every corner of the planet. There is an old aphorism: "What you see is what you get." On a metaphysical level, this has potent implications. Thoughts have tremendous energy. In this instance, our visualization serves two purposes. First, when we think differently about something, we also treat it differently. So, positive visualization leads to affirmative action. Secondly, each time we imagine the Earth's wholeness, our thoughts send out beneficial vibrations to affect that wholeness.

HELPFUL HINTS

If you are involved in healing, you are already, in some way, Gaia's servant, for you aid her children. Beyond that, if you would like to do more to help global healing, here are some simple ways for anyone, anywhere, to begin:

Coordinate regular meetings among like-minded citizens to offer new ideas, support, and enthusiasm to each other. Have each member of this group bring pertinent articles that keep everyone aware and informed. Write letters to your regional leaders and vote for Earth-first politicians. Support any local programs your community may offer.

Educate yourself. Knowledge unlocks many doors, and learning about ecology and recycling is not that difficult these days. In the process, you will find that you can also save a lot of money by creative reuse of items you once threw out. Just check your local library for books—sometimes the ones that include children's projects are the best (even for adults). They are simple, forthright, and practical for our busy society.

As you're doing your other spiritual work, take a moment out and send energy back to the Earth. Every time we work in metaphysical realms, we draw on universal energy, of which the Earth is part. Reciprocity means that we don't take this power for granted, but return the favor!

When you're walking outdoors, sing, chant, or play uplifting Earth-centered songs. Plants and animals both benefit from sacred songs and words, as will you. There are hundreds of wonderful CDs and tapes you can get with music that stimulates a One-World mindset and honors nature.

Don't overlook simple gestures. If you have an extra crystal, bless it and return it to the Earth. If you can buy a 59¢ package of seeds, toss them into an open field or your own back yard to generate new plants or flowers. Extend love to the things you grow in and around your home. Since all living things are connected to the Earth, loving one tree is loving the whole planet (think globally)!

Consider the impact of everything you do. For example, if everyone decreased their meat consumption by 10 percent, we could provide 12 million tons of grain for human or animal consumption annually.[8]

Live as simply as possible, use Earth-friendly products and technology, and change your way of thinking to a conservative, preservative approach.

As you begin your efforts, remember that each blade of grass, each flower, and each creature is an integral part of the ecosystem network. So even the smallest efforts for global healing can have far-reaching effects. Don't feel that you have to change the world overnight; just change little pieces of it one day at a time. It is actually much more appropriate to begin Earth-healing efforts in your own back yard. Each person, changing personal habits and values where they live, is essential if we ever hope to see far-reaching results.

Technology can be our servant, not our master. We can find the sacredness in everyone and everything by using the right eyes and the proper attitude. Ecospirituality reminds us that the way we approach something changes its function. So when we approach our environment as hallowed (even if it's a city), it becomes hallowed. St. Benedict understood this principle, when he said to regard "all utensils and goods of the monastery as sacred vessels of the altar."[9]

---

[8]Andrew Robbins, *Diet for a New America* (Walpole, NH: Stillpoint Publishing, 1987), p. 352.
[9]Charles Cummings, "Benedictine Reverence Revisited," *American Benedictine Review, 41:3*, 1990, p. 325.

Eventually, the path of reverence leads to a communion with creation that is powerful and transformational. It inspires love of all living things, love of god, and love of self. The lesson of Gaia's healers can be found in love; for it is truly this energy combined with hands-on effort that brings wholeness.

9

Elemental Healing

*All the arts lose virtue against the essential
reality of creatures going about their business
among the equally earnest elements of nature.*

—Robinson Jeffers

NUMEROUS ANCIENT PHILOSOPHIES DISCUSSED
the elements in connection with human health and wellness, as well as spirituality. One of the best examples comes
from the 1500s with an alchemist named Dr. Sigismund
Bacstrom. Dr. Bacstrom wrote that, if all the elements could
be united into a stone, symbolically represented by two in-
terlaced triangles, this token would give the bearer the
power to heal all sickness.

The ancient Greeks characterized the elements by specific shapes, as did Cabalists. By combining these symbols
with other healing methods like visualization, an elemental
healer can achieve improved results (see Table 5, p. 167).
For example, a massage therapist may add a guided visualization wherein typically flighty patients envision themselves in a cube of white-green light to improve their foundations.

Today, "bodywork" is a term denoting schools of holistic therapy that increase a patient's awareness of the
elemental self for the purpose of improved health. (See
Table 5 on page 167.) Chiropractors and osteopaths, for example, use physical manipulation that adjusts the body so it

Table 5. Elements, Associated Symbols, and Shapes.

ELEMENT	CABALISTIC SYMBOL	GREEK SHAPE
Water	▽	Icosahedral
Air	△ (with line)	Octahedral as an intermediary between water and fire
Fire	△	Tetrahedral
Earth	▽ (with line)	Cubical for stability
Spirit	△ (with inner triangle)	n/a
Source	(circled star symbol)	Dodecahedron as the mingling of all elements and matrix of the universe.

handles living with the Earth element more effectively—
e.g. these adjustments often provide patients with a change
in their center of gravity so they learn to walk, sit, and stand
correctly, working *with* Earth's gravity, instead of against it.

Similarly, rolfing releases stress and tension from coping with the world, but is centered on the emotional
instead of the physical struggle with gravity. Thus, rolfing
is considered a water-centered healing technique, this
element being more strongly attuned to the emotional
disposition.

Air is part of nearly all alternative therapies, relating
directly to the patient's breathing pattern. For more information on breath, refer to the section on guided meditation and visualization. Finally, the fire element is magnet-
ism, upon which acupressure, Reiki, and some massage
therapies focus.

Actually, all healing has an elemental nature. Fire purifies, water soothes, air refreshes, and earth dispels. So its
not surprising to discover that each element can play an ef-

fective role in the creative healer's kit beyond those mentioned above.

EARTH

In the Bible, Earth was the seed of creation: the very genesis of humankind. The Plains Indians revere the Earth as the beginning and end of all life. Slavic people swear oaths on the soil, and ask the Earth to bear witness to their conviction. During times of plague, early Russians held processionals, digging furrows in the Earth so its spirit could emerge to fight for their people. Effectively, what each of these diverse cultural traditions tells us is that the Earth gave us birth, and therefore can certainly help us maintain wellness.

Soil has a nurturing, fertile quality. It represents stable ground, receptivity, and maturity within the natural order of time. Earth's gravity, specifically, exercises a drawing power—similar to the way magnets were used in early healing rituals to "extract" sickness.

Hands-on healers who choose the earth element as their focus may use salt, clay, rocks, holed stones, iron, lead, seeds, wheat, or acorns as just a few of their tools. Realistically, the earth-healer may choose any natural item with which to work, as it all reconnects to Gaia. Additionally, earth-centered techniques can be accented by coordinating them with the astrological signs of Taurus, Virgo, and Capricorn. Here are some examples of specific forms of elemental earth healing:

Clay: Especially good for cleansing and toning skin; red clay helps draw out toxins, such as those from insect bites; yellow clay purifies; green clays are useful in many forms of healing. For some treatments, the clay may be warmed to increase effectiveness.

Warm sand for joint conditions: From a purely logical perspective, this feels quite comforting. The warmth helps ease pain.

Soil, sand, or clay burials: This is like a mock death, where the patient literally and figuratively emerges as a new being. Alternatively, when patients can not participate, poppets might take their place, filled with symbolic herbs and clothed with a piece of personal fabric.

Holed stones—Passing through: In Cornwall, there stands a huge Menantol that people regularly used in healing rites. Here, patients were passed through the rock to mark the passage from sickness to health. Similar to soil burials, this also seemed symbolically to indicate a new life—one free of disease.

Stones buried in the ground: Among South Africans, a painted stone placed in the entryway of a village protected the entire region from plague.

Dust: When found beneath a stone where two roads met, dust was once thought quite potent for healing warts. An inflicted person would rub the warts with the dust, then disperse it to the winds (England). Dust from a graveyard was also a potent curative for many years, because it symbolized power over death. The latent energy in this emblem also has something to do with the fact that graveyards are sanctified ground. Any region regarded as holy is considered doubly effective from a folk healer's perspective.

WATER

In Finno-Ugric traditions, the Tonx spirit and the *VuKutis* (another water spirit) both had the power to overcome sickness and fight disease. Babylonians regarded water as an instrument of the gods' justice, and Greek water nymphs were purported to heal the sick if asked properly. For an ancient Slavonic sect known as Kupalu, water was a mystical power worthy of worship. Before the Kupalu's festivals, all followers washed in rivers, then honored sacred springs and wells with prayers and offerings.

Metaphysically, water cleanses, soothes, flows, and receives. It encompasses the gentle sounds of waves that carry all-important rest and sleep. Water energies are accented by the astrological signs of Pisces, Scorpio, and Cancer. Symbolically, mercury, silver, copper, ice, snow, fog, shells, and the season of Autumn all embody its potency.

As with fire and the Sun, elemental water-healing cannot be totally divorced from lunar influences. The oceans and lakes follow the Moon's energy, rising and falling at its bidding. Among people in northern regions, particularly the Norse people, tides had great significance—those especially helpful to healing being midnight tides for health, premorning tides for rest and recuperation, midday tides for fortitude, and predusk tides for transformation.

Soaking or washing in sea water: Among the Scots, washing a patient's hands and feet three times, then pouring the left-over water on the hearth was an ancient charm to break sickness' domain.

Travel to sacred fonts and wells: Once people arrived at a region like Lourdes, they often walked around the area three times and offered the indwelling spirit food, beverages, or coins. Our modern tradition of making wishes at a well is based on this ancient custom.

Sweet water rinse: Being pure and totally safe for consumption, sweet water has been recommended to release negativity and bring joy to someone who is ailing.

Cupped hands of water: Besides being a rite for rain, water tossed overhead thrice can help change auric energy. This approach is shamanic in origins.

Singing or speaking sacred words to water: If you can't reach someone, convey wellness with a wave. Think back to your days in Earth Science where you learned about water's cycle. It not only moves out from you on the crest, but also goes into the air, so your energy can bless the Earth as it travels to its destination.

A Gift from Karl

Several years ago when I was having a particularly trying day, I went out to our front porch, not wanting my son to see me so upset. He followed me, saw my tears, and began crying. Through that veil of water he said, "Don't be sad, Mommy." The purity of his love and caring touched me deeply. In a moment of inspiration, I wiped his face, put his tears in my glass of water, and internalized that pure love by drinking the water. This seemed to be the perfect element to convey that profound emotion, allowing compassionate energy to flow direct to my heart where it was most needed.

FIRE

Ancient Persians had a cult centered around fire as the ultimate principle of light, purity, and life. Its ability to drive away the darkness made the Sun (a ball of fire) the most popular object to eventually develop divine status among early peoples throughout the Earth. In India, for example, Ushas is a god of dawn who brings life and health to all things.

The theme of fire's importance and potency is repeated again and again in numerous cultures. From Japan to Scotland, special festivals were held to dispense hearth fire so that entire communities could live well and warmly for the coming year. Here, fire equated to the heart of a home, love, unity, and continued sustenance.

Fire represents purification and total renewal. Like the phoenix rising from its ashes, fire forcefully banishes and protects. Its tokens include the colors red, orange, and bright blue, lava stone, gold, brass, any fire source, and noontime, when shadows must flee. It is accented by the signs of Aries, Leo, and Sagittarius.

Ashes from sacred fires: Considered as already accepted by the Divine, these ashes are akin to those used for anointing on Ash Wednesday. Usually, however, ritual ashes get used for earth or animal healing. For the former, the ashes get sprinkled on, or mingled with, the soil. For a creature, they might be brushed into the fur or put into a bed cushion.

Fire diagnosis: Some fire healers take their patients to a remote spot and ask them to build a fire. They use the final construction of this fire as a tool for diagnosis.

Candle: Burn the image of a problem away in the flame of a red candle. After you are done, let the candle burn out, likewise extinguishing the malady.

Poppet: Burn the image of sickness. Alternatively, ancient Babylonians consigned clay images to the fire to consume the difficulty.

Fires: Scottish witches passed sickly children over the flames of a small fire, "thrice to the other side," marking a new beginning beyond the reach of illness. Similarly, in England, people were conveyed over a small bramble fire seven times, the number representing completion. For our purposes, a candle flame might be a safer alternative.

AIR

Among the ancient Greeks and Phoenicians, breath was considered the first-born of two great principles, even before the advent of the Cosmic Egg. This may explain the use of wind as an essential element in the oracle at Donada. In Japanese beliefs, the wind god resides between the Earth and the Heavens, filling the void therein. The Bible speaks of the creative breath of God and, among Tibetan monks, sand paintings are dispersed reverently to the winds to help heal the Earth.

Air is an element of freshness, movement, and freedom—all potent symbols for healing. It is strongly associated with the season of Spring and dawn. Both these times are perfect for new beginnings—beginnings that are filled with healthy bodies!

Air healers may choose to fan someone with cleansing herbs or open the windows of a sickroom to refresh the whole house. Practically speaking, this last action also helps to keep germs from breeding. Other symbols and items useful to air-healers include tin or copper, the astrological signs of Gemini, Libra, or Aquarius, feathers, and flowers.

Symbols on the wind for change: Since wind is an element with movement, scattering light items on the winds to emblematically convey health to someone, or transport sickness away, seems appropriate. Try to choose an item that won't harm wildlife or the planet in any way—dry dirt being one possibility (see also earth-healing, this chapter). In this instance, the patient should hold the soil, visualizing their malady pouring into it, then cast the dirt to the wind to disperse negative energy.

Directional winds: It is good to know that the air has a way of allowing us to touch the other three elements just by changing direction. Southerly winds are fire, westerly winds are water, and northerly winds have the element earth mingled therein. Consequently, combining healing with a specific directional wind can empower the effort further. For example, if working with patients suffering from a lack of energy, you might want to give them an invigorating rubdown in the presence of a southerly wind for increased vitality.

Flowers for the infirm: Why do we take flowers to sick people? Certainly this has something to do with flowers' beauty. The art of aromatherapy should not be discounted as a partial answer to this question either! Many ancient herbalists discussed the virtues of a flower's scent to aid emotional distress. Carried on gentle breezes, a flower's aroma has the capacity to improve a patient's temperament, thereby speeding the recuperative process.

Tickle me well: Feathers are an excellent symbol of air. In modern magical circles, a priest or priestess might be seen bearing a feather and incense with which to smudge participants—e.g., fan away any sickness or negativity with the feather, the smoke conveying it on the winds. A technique similar to this one can be adapted to a patient's aura without the use of incense. In this instance, the healer uses a feather to tickle the aura, sensitively moving any contrary energy away, and bringing renewed happiness with each stroke.

ELEMENTAL BLENDS

In nature, the elements rarely work alone. Theirs is a concert of harmonious cooperation. Consequently, healers who learn how to apply or adapt more than one element in their work generally discover improved success rates. The reason for this is not only the increased power afforded by the presence of other elements, but also the fact that each patient responds to each element differently. So, elemental healers who combine symbols and tools have a better chance of striking that perfect symmetry with a patient that begins the path to wholeness. Here are some potential examples of effective combinations:

Sand as combination of fire/earth or water/earth: This depends mostly on where the healer gathers the sand. If from the desert, it is fire/earth (and perhaps a little water).

Damp sea breeze as water/air: To collect this, leave a dry cotton cloth hung over a clean frame at sundown for several hours (or just before sunrise) and squeeze out the dew. There is additional symbolism gained here in either choice of timing. Sunset marks an ending and a time of rest. Just before sunrise anticipates a new beginning after sickness passes.

Woodash as fire/earth: Recommended for external use only, and then only to regions that don't exhibit rashes or open cuts that could become infected.

Incense as fire/air: See "Tickle me well," this chapter.

Mud as earth/water: Beauticians still use mudpacks, and in fact, certain types of mud with high mineral content are much sought after by the cosmetic industry. All the elemental healer is doing here is invoking a positive latent energy!

Steam as fire/water: Most practically used to help those with congestion. Add some refreshing herbs to boiling water and have patients breathe deeply. Take care that patients close their eyes and don't get too close to the hot water, however. Steaming is also good for sore muscles and general relaxation. For most people, this can be achieved at home simply by running just the hot water in a shower for a while with the bathroom door closed.

Elemental healing is easily applied to any other methods discussed herein, and is one of the easiest techniques for everyone to learn. Generally, the source material for elemental healing is folk medicine, where everything that could potentially improve a patient's physical, mental, or spiritual well-being was tried at least once, especially when conventional methods failed. Thus, many of the "remedials" spoken of here may seem a little antiquated. Nonetheless, they still reflect the holistic attitude that all hands-on healers should develop—the attitude that searches out the best possible avenue to improve a patient's quality of living.

10

Flower Remedies

To see a world in a Grain of Sand,
And a Heaven in a Wild Flower . . .
—William Blake

AS WITH AROMAS, OUR FOREFATHERS KNEW THAT
nature's pharmacopeia was diverse and useful, including
substances from flowers. Hippocrates, Pliny, Culpepper,
and other well-known herbalists recommended flowers regularly as remedials, the most popular of which was the rose.
Similarly, for emotional problems in the 17th century, bor-
age was taken to provide a fearful patient with improved
fortitude and determination.

Despite the popularity of flowers in herbalism and
cooking up through the early 1900s, it took the efforts of a
London physician to bring flowers solidly into the field of
homeopathy. In the 1930s, Dr. Edward Bach left a very lu-
crative medical practice as a bacteriologist in England to try
and find other ways to help his patients. Dr. Bach felt that
most disease was caused by mental distress and anxiety,
which lowers the body's resistance. In his studies, he noted
that ailing animals often lick the dew from flowers. From
this simple lesson of nature, he eventually formulated the
Bach Flower Remedies, which consist of 38 different flower-
based curatives aimed at emotional problems that exhibit
themselves through physical symptoms.

To make the flower remedies, Dr. Bach insisted that the flowers be picked at the height of their bloom, on a sunny day, from an uncultivated area. The remedies are prepared very quickly thereafter so no potency is lost. This is done by infusing the flowers in water out in the sunshine. This liquid is preserved in an alcohol base and used as a tincture. The FDA approved Bach's remedies for public sale as a homeopathic treatment, even though there is little documentation regarding their efficacy.

Flower remedies use the ideas of vibrational medicine as their foundation. To paraphrase Dr. Bach, the remedies raise the vibration of our spirits, and, by so doing, eliminate the lower ranges of energy within which disease can abide. Everything in this universe has a unique pattern or matrix, at least part of which mirrors the originating source. When our basic matrix energy increases, we come closer to that source. In the presence of such power, sickness cannot endure.

Many philosophers have thought that nature was the most perfect reflection of the Originating Source. In Eastern belief systems especially, flowers symbolize spiritual potential and development. Dr. Bach just took this idea a little further—by distilling the essence of positive spiritual attributes in flowers and finding a way for those characteristics to blossom in the human psyche. Medically speaking, when a patient consumes the flower essences, transformation begins on the circulatory level, then moves into the nervous system and eventually into the meridians and chakras.

Dr. Bach believed that everyone already has sparks of positive characteristics within their soul matrix. The flower essences, therefore, shake up that latent energy and get it moving functionally into daily living. The remedies become catalysts for rediscovering harmony and wholeness. None of the remedies are "carved in stone," however, since each individual reacts differently depending on development, openness, and sensitivity. See Table 6 on page 180.

Table 6. BACH REMEDIES (abbreviated).

PROBLEM/EMOTION	ESSENCE	RESULT
Adjustment (difficult)	Walnut	Acclimation
Anxiety (severe)	Sweet chestnut	Tranquility
Apathy	Wild rose	Zeal
Apprehension	Aspen	Dauntlessness
Arrogance	Water violet	Balanced humility
Bitterness	Willow	Congeniality
Chronic fatigue	Olive	Composure, peace
Cycle repetitions	Chestnut bud	Breaking habits
Daydreaming, Inattentiveness	Clematis	Alertness, grounded
Dejection	Sweet chestnut	Renewed faith
Depression	Mustard	Self-confidence
Dissatisfaction	Wild oat	Clear ambitions
Despondency	Gorse	Hope
Distraction, Restlessness	Agrimony	Composure
Distraction, Restlessness	White chestnut	Concentration
Domination	Vine	Delegation
Emotional explosiveness	Cherry plum	Calm nerves
Exhaustion (mental)	Hornbeam	Vitality
Extroversion (extreme)	Heather	Sensitivity
Facades (carefree)	Agrimony	Sincerity
Fanaticism	Vervain	Equilibrium
Fantasizing	Clematis	Grounded reasoning
Fear, panic attacks	Rock rose	Courage
Fear, panic attacks	Aspen	Security
Emotional suppression	Beech	Openness, release
Exhaustion (body/mind)	Olive	Vitality
Guilt	Pine	Candor, peace
Haste	Impatiens	Forbearance
Idealism	Crab apple	Practicality
Incompetence (perceived)	Elm	Trust
Indecisiveness	Scleranthus	Conclusiveness
Inferiority complex	Larch	Self-reliance
Inflexibility	Vine	Wise leadership
Intolerance, Judgment	Beech	Acceptance
Jealousy	Holly	Universal love
Listlessness	Wild oat	Ambition
Manipulativeness	Chicory	Acceptance
Melancholy, gloom	Mustard	Serenity
Misgivings, phobias	Oak	Stability, hope
Overzealousness	Vervain	Paced energy

Table 6. BACH REMEDIES continued.		
PROBLEM/EMOTION	ESSENCE	RESULT
Pessimism	Gorse	Renewed faith
Post-traumatic stress	Star of Bethlehem	Recovery
Prejudice	Beech	Impartiality
Procrastination	Hornbeam	Expediency
Reactive (excessively)	Impatiens	Composure
Rigidity	Rock water	Open-mindedness
Self-doubt	Cerato	Confidence
Selfishness	Chicory	Generosity
Self-sacrifice	Centaury	Self-fulfillment
Sentimentality	Honeysuckle	Releasing the past
Shyness/Timidity	Mimulus	Boldness
Skepticism	Gentian	Faith, optimism
Sloth	Wild rose	Renewed vitality
Subservience	Centaury	Assurance
Temper out of control	Cherry plum	Self-regulation
Unyielding to exhaustion	Oak	Endurance, common sense
Vacillation (decisions)	Scleranthus	Resolution
Wavering convictions	Walnut	Determination
Withdrawal	Water violet	Sociability
Worry	White chestnut	Acceptance
Worry	Red chestnut	Positive outlook

In diagnosing a problem or condition, several steps are followed. First, healers should not begin working until they've reached a centered, calm state of awareness. Secondly, the prescription should not be a matter of logic, but of insight. Interview the patient to get information on tensions, fears, feelings, and symptoms. From this interview, and perhaps by adding other diagnostic techniques like dowsing (alongside a healthy portion of knowing human behavior), the healer then decides upon a course of therapy.

A Bach therapy session can last anywhere from 40 to 60 minutes because of the observation and discussion involved. There is no pat answer for when to change a therapy or how long a treatment should continue. This is due to the individualized, intuitive nature of this holistic approach. About the only "rule" that the Bach Center really advocates is that a patient should use a maximum of six or seven therapies consecutively (returning to the homeopathic idea of less being more). Bach's flower therapy may also be used on animals and children.

Dr. Bach recommended that people who learned his therapies first spend a year getting to know the remedies and their effects on themselves. He also felt it was very important that healers not allow personal fears, prejudices, or repressive ideas to distort their perceptions of others' needs. This writer feels that he had two excellent points, well worth applying to other types of healing approaches as well!

Bach was not the only person to study and develop flower therapies. Richard Katz and his wife Patricia Kaminski founded the Flower Essence Society in California for the purpose of networking with other people around the world who utilize flower therapies. This group also researches new remedials, conducts classes, and holds retreats. As of 1986, there were 72 flower essences recommended by the Society for specific emotional categories.

Another healer, by the name of Gurudas, wrote about 108 new flower essences (some of which are included in the Society's work) in *Flower Essences and Vibrational Healing* (1983). Kevin Ryerson, a predominant channeler and member of the Association for Research and Enlightenment helped devise these listings through his channeling skills. These people, like Bach, believe that illness reflects a disharmony between the personality and the higher self. This causes imbalanced energy patterns throughout the body and aura to which the essences are applied, rather as a mechanic uses tools to realign automobile tires!

Last, but not least, the art of flower therapy should not be totally divorced from that of aromatherapy. While the two approaches are different in application, both depend on natural extracts and both rely on vibrational cues for success. Whether or not flower remedies have any verifiable effect probably matters little, since they are safe even by FDA standards. Since Dr. Bach advocated the idea of self-healing, just taking the step to obtain the flower remedies is a positive action. This means patients have recognized deficiencies in themselves, want to make a change, and are taking steps to do just that! Any psychologist will be happy to confirm that acknowledgment, honest desire, and affirmative action represent the most important elements to improving your emotional state. For more information on Bach remedies and other flower essence remedies you can contact the following:

The Bach Center
Mount Vernon
Sotwell, Wallingford
Oxon OX10 0PZ,
England
Phone: 011-44-1491-834-678
Fax: 011-44-1491-825-022
E-Mail: centre@bachcentre.com
www.bachcentre.com

Global Health Alternatives
193 Middle St. #281
Portland, ME 04104
1-800-4BECALM

Flower Essence Pharmacy
2007 Northeast 39th Ave.
Portland, OR 97212
1-800-343-8693
Fax: 503-284-7090

11

Food and Fitness

Every man is the builder of a temple,
called his body . . .
—Henry David Thoreau

IN REVIEWING CONTEMPORARY TRENDS, IT SEEMS as if nearly everyone has jumped on the food and fitness bandwagon. Hundreds of people, many of whom are famous, have special "work out" videos to keep us slim, trim, and physically fit. Others write diet guides and cookbooks to help with everything from heart trouble to sexual deficiencies.[1] Not all of these individuals write from a New Age outlook, but most agree that we do not treat our bodies with the respect due them.

In nearly every metaphysical tradition, the body is considered the temple of the soul—a housing within which the immutable essence of our true self grows and learns. If the foundation of this house is shaky, our spiritual roots are likewise insecure. When the windows are dirty, our spiritual vision becomes clouded. When the stairs or floors are in disrepair, our spiritual footing is similarly uncertain.

---

[1] In all fairness, I must confess that I am among this number with *Kitchen Witch's Cookbook* (St. Paul, MN: Llewellyn, 1995). However, the ultimate intention of this title was to add a little spiritual energy to food versus changing people's diets.

Wellness is more than just the absence of disease. It includes self-awareness and self-love manifested through how we treat our bodies. Because our nature is threefold, care and attention toward the physical self will positively affect the spiritual and mental. The antithesis is also true.

Our feelings about what we eat and about our physical nature influence metaphysical energies. How often have you known people who do not like their external image to be depressed or sick regularly? Such individuals are also less likely to have confidence in their spiritual vision, thereby undermining the positive energy in and around their lives.

Similarly, people with fast-paced lifestyles that allow little time for nutritional food and fitness programs often show signs of stress-related syndromes. The end result is an imbalance that manifests physically as weariness, sore muscles, colds, heartburn, and other maladies. Spiritually, this can exhibit itself as a blocked flow of energy, closed chakras, and harsh auric fields (just to name a few).

So those involved in New Age food and fitness teachings are simply trying to remind us that we need to take care of ourselves. They remind us that physical awareness and personal care is part of "enlightenment" too. Without this part of the equation, the cauldron of our being is lopsided, trying to balance on two legs instead of the three that provide stability.

FOOD

Foods and beverages have played a key role throughout history. Even our earliest ancestors gathered together for "dinner." All manner of foods and beverages appeared on altars to the Gods. The Celts drank from communal cups to show their unity, while in England, a King's cup was likened to

the Grail. Folk healers used certain foods for their curatives, notably potatoes for warts.

While it may seem that we are far away from such a
world, in truth, our daily eating and drinking "rituals"
speak loudly of this past. We consume certain items pas-
sionately (like hot fudge sundaes), others we loudly detest.
People who enjoy cooking may zealously guard their favorite cookware and recipes with as much seriousness as
any holy items. People who love coffee guard their favorite
drinking mug! Couples at a wedding still frequently drink
from one glass during the ceremony to symbolically link
their destinies, and my mother rubbed potatoes on burns
and warts. All these nonchalant actions have their foundations in much earlier times.

Some foods remind us of special events, others are cul-
turally or religiously significant. Then there are "family"
foods that become an integral part of gathering with kin.
Thus, the effect of tradition cannot be ignored by dietary
counselors—it is perhaps as powerful a tool for achieving
wholeness as proper nutritional values. For example, what
happens if we encourage people to eat something they consider "taboo?" This food might be the right prescription for
physical health, but the mental impact is very detrimental.
This is true to the extent that it could result in *real* dis-ease!

The moral of the story? Treat every portion of your existence with equal respect and attention, and the result will
be the most productive spiritual life for which you can
hope.

A HISTORY OF NUTRITION

At the turn of the century, mothers everywhere strove to
serve good food to their families. They did not fret over
how much meat or potato was included in that diet—as
long as it filled the stomach, tasted good, and provided en-

ergy, the meal was successful. Does this mean that our current emphasis on nutrition and diet is something new? Not at all.

Hippocrates (400 B.C.), considered the father of medicine, indicated an interest in dietary studies for improved health, as did Galen (A.D. 200), a fellow Grecian physician and philosopher. Between the fifth century B.C. and the first century A.D., a famous Indian physician named Charaka developed Ayurvedic medicine. Charaka ascribed a great deal of importance to his patients' diets. This form of healing alters food intake to restore balance to the body's *dosha*, or vital energy.

Taking a leap forward to the Middle Ages, a 16th-century Italian doctor named Sanctorius[2] did extensive work on diet. Sanctorius went so far as to weigh his food, weigh himself before and after eating, and weigh excretions to see how much food his body was using. His notes meticulously cover thirty years of such arduous examination.

A contemporary of Sanctorius, Paracelsus, was taking a slightly different approach, that of dietary prescriptions. When a well-known scholar named Forben became critically ill with an infected leg. Paracelsus gave strict orders to his cook. No rich foods or wines, simple meals, and plenty of juice, herbal teas, or broths. Six days later, Forben was well enough to go walking, and thanked Paracelsus by recommending he be appointed the city physician for Basel.

A 17th-century Tibetan medical treatise illustrates the four disciplines for good health as nutrition, lifestyle, medicines and herbs, and external treatments.[3] The first two of these could be regulated by the individual, but the other two came from healer/ministers in the community. At this

---

[2]Elmer V. McCollum, *History of Nutrition* (Boston, MA: Houghton Mifflin, 1957).

[3]Time-Life Books eds. *Powers of Healing* (Alexandria, VA: Time-Life Books, 1989), p. 63.

early juncture, we must remember that many priests, in various cultures, were also healers.

From these examples, it is obvious that we are not the first people on this planet to examine our eating patterns. Thanks to modern forms of communication, however, information on diet and nutrition is far more available to us than it was to our ancestors. Thus, it is also more popularized.

For example, a 1995 article from the Wall Street Journal[4] reported that Darwinian medicine is showing signs of growth. Darwinians believe that studying the way our ancestors lived and what they ate will help us rediscover nutritional and physical balance today. Basically, the founding concept behind this school of thought is that medical science often overlooks the evolutionary changes that have shaped people when recommending treatment or diet.

Darwinians recommend things like staying away from aspirin, antinausea drugs during pregnancy, and iron supplements when you are ill. Sound crazy? Even Darwinians agree that their ideas are controversial, but that's the whole point. They want to get people asking questions that haven't been adequately addressed by modern medicine. Included in this list is exactly how and why we get sick!

Apparently our ancestral patterns aren't quite equipped to handle life's pace these days. Genetic codes developed over hundreds of thousands of years. In the last century, the entire velocity of human existence has drastically increased. This is certainly not enough time for adequate genetic adaptation.

Our ancestors lived much simpler lives than we, eating little or no dairy products, some game meat (which is low-fat), and hefty amounts of grains, fruits, and vegetables. This diet resulted in lower cholesterol levels than that of

---

[4] *Wall Street Journal*, Vol. LXXVI, No. 155, p. A1, A6.

the average person today. They also ate calcium-rich greens like broccoli regularly, giving the total Stone Age menu about 20 percent of its calories from fat, one-half that of the American diet!

CONTEMPORARY EATING HABITS

Benjamin Franklin once said that "one should eat to live, not live to eat." Most New Age dietary teachers agree with this philosophy. While not all lecture us on the evils of sugar and fat, they do encourage more thoughtfulness in our cooking and eating habits. They also remind us that we should cook and eat with a loving, grateful heart to help internalize the most positive aspects of our meals.[5]

With this last idea in mind, revitalizing the tradition of meal-time prayers may be long overdue! Prayers are focused thoughts (like meditations or spells) that extend energy for a specific purpose—that of health and vitality. They also take time out of our rushing to thank the Earth and the Great Spirit for their providence, something Native Americans have always done.

Modern dietary consultants recognize that we live in a very hectic world where all of us, at one time or another, skip meals or eat whatever is expedient. If this continues regularly for a few weeks, we become too sick or weary to do anything productive. When the physical nature gets ignored, sickness or exhaustion is our body's cry for attention.[6]

Thus, people in this field encourage us to slow down a bit. They remind us to eat somewhat balanced meals whenever possible and pay close attention to the signals our

---

[5]Joan Borysenko, *Minding Our Bodies, Mending the Mind* (Reading, MA: Addison-Wesley, 1987).
[6]Jane Brody, *Jane Brody's Nutrition Book* (New York: Bantam, 1987).

bodies provide. A craving for an unusual food (not chocolate), for example, can be the body's way of expressing what it needs. When a healthy diet is not possible, ask a holistician, herbalist, or pharmacist for a daily supplement.

The number of approaches to sound eating is almost overwhelming. Herbalists have made us more aware of the wonders of nature's pantry, stuffed full with nutritional value (see also chapter 12). Here, a wealth of options for cooking and personal enrichment present themselves unwittingly disguised as roots, leaves, flowers, and trees. Vitamin experts detail the warning signs of problems and the proper foods to balance them out. Some experts report that a symmetry of acidity and alkaline content is important to our physiology, while others recommend abstaining from meat.

No matter the stricture, certain New Age dietary guidelines do appear to be somewhat universal.[7] Here are just a few:

> Being well fed does not necessarily mean being well nourished. Nourishment, by definition, implies taking in substances necessary to life and growth.

> Decrease the amount of red meat in our diets; the meats that we do consume should be properly handled and thoroughly cooked.

> Soy sauce is an excellent substitute for salt as it supplies enzymes. Yogurt, sauerkraut, and pickles also provide this essential ingredient to our diet. Best taken twice a week.[8]

---

[7]Two excellent books that cover this topic are *Natural Healing* by Marcia Stark (St. Paul, MN: Llewellyn, 1991) and *Earthway* by Mary Summer Rain (New York: Pocket Books, 1990).

[8]Michio Kushi, *The Book of Macrobiotics: The Universal Way of Health and Happiness* (Tokyo: Japan Publications, 1977).

Moderation is a key to success. For example, whole grains provide complex carbohydrates that maintain blood sugar. Thus cereal is great in the morning, but should not be consumed later in the evening for best digestion and sleep patterns.

If you crave sugar, eat a natural sugar (like fruit or nut seeds).

Eating a good variety in your foods can help avoid allergies. Also, certain foods in combination produce essential amino acids.

If you're struggling with obesity, eat slowly, savor your food, and don't eat in front of the TV. Avoid snacking between meals, drink a glass of water before eating, lower your salt intake and eat approximately two tablespoons of fiber daily. Allow yourself a few treats weekly with appropriate moderation, and start a slow, progressive exercise program. These steps combined with improved self-images will help control this difficulty.

Stay away from artificial colors, sweeteners, and fruits and vegetables grown with herbicides. Vine ripened food is more nutrient rich.

In terms of cooking, frying is the worst for us physically; braise or broil instead. Steaming vegetables produces the highest content of vitamins and minerals upon consumption.

Take care in the cleanliness of your food preparation items and eating utensils. Wash all surfaces thoroughly with soap and water before and after food preparation. Avoid wooden cutting boards to decrease germs.

Refrain from cooking and eating when you are tense, ill, angry, or otherwise out of sorts. This not only affects digestion, but that negative energy can be transferred into food.

Limit your intake of alcohol, and drink plenty of water. If the water in your region is bad, buy spring water or get a water filter.

Rinse poultry, fruits, and vegetables before you cook them. Also wash the lids on cans and bottles before opening to remove any dust and dirt.

Whenever possible, take your time eating. Thank the founder of your feast and enjoy the food.

Any foods that are left out for general consumption should have proper coverings to keep away flies, pets, and unwanted dirt.

If you're having trouble with weight gain or loss, consult a professional, not a "quick fix" guru. Diet pills can be very dangerous, as can be the best-intentioned advice.

Include vegetable juices, broths, and herbal teas in your diet daily to help improve digestion and toxin elimination.

Never refreeze foods and remember the basic kitchen motto: *When in doubt, throw it out!*[9]

A final note: some dietary counselors suggest that we refrain from eating anything that we wouldn't place upon the

---

[9]I hate to waste food, but being frugal does not require that you get sick in the process. Store your leftovers properly and cook only what you need and the instances of waste will decrease.

altar as an offering. This idea left me pondering for weeks over its significance. During ancient times, our forbears gave of their abundance to the gods—and it was food from their own tables. As they fed the divine, the leftovers went to worshippers, which acted as a silent acknowledgement of the "god" within each person.

Could we comfortably give our god/dess a burger, fries, and a cola? If not, then I must ask myself why people (including myself) continue to give their inner "god" similar items. I can't honestly say that I have an answer on this subject. Nonetheless it is certainly "food for thought."

For more information on foods, their safety, labeling, and proper handling instructions, call the U.S. Agriculture Hotline: 1-800-535-4555 or write Consumer Information Center, Pueblo, CO 81009.

EXERCISE

Many ancient Western cultures valued athletic skill and physical bearing. One need only look at the Roman and Mayan games and Greek sculpture to verify this. The Greeks in particular elevated fitness to a lofty goal that was part of individual development. Among Eastern peoples, the martial arts evolved as an expression of both philosophical ideals and physical conditioning.

No matter the location, all of these activities honed the bodies of the participants. Some of the pastimes also venerated higher spiritual concepts—in Greece, that of beauty; in China, that of placement; in certain Native American tribes, that of acknowledging the Great Spirit's presence. This approach is exactly what New Age exercise teachers hope to rekindle—aiding the body while improving the mind and expanding the spirit.

Physical exertion was a natural activity for our ancestors. It wasn't something they had to fit into their schedule.

At the time of Christ, the primary occupations were herding and hunting. By the 1400s, the focus changed to agriculture. Even in the 1800s around 90 percent of the population was agrarian, meaning most people had a very rigorous daily routine centered around their homes and farms.

In the last one hundred years, however, the focus of our society has shifted from physical to mental labor, meaning many people have no defined daily activity other than sitting at a desk. This lack of exercise can have many negative outcomes including increased tension, digestive disorders, heart problems, and a tendency to fatigue easily. Additionally, inactivity can foster depression and decrease one's resistance to disease.

Exactly what brought about the fitness trend in modern culture is uncertain. In part, the labor-saving devices that have left some people overweight and lazy are certainly one part of the picture. Additionally, when medicine became available to the vast majority of the populace, the knowledge of the hazards of unfit bodies spread. The New Age movement is also playing a vital role in turning people's attention back to the sacredness of the body.

All of these factors combine to form what has become a modern fad. Exercise is chic and trendy. One can buy all types of exercise equipment and clothing just about everywhere. This is not necessarily bad, unless taken to extremes by those trying to live up to unrealistic images. Fitness does not equate to outward attractiveness, yet that is how it's being sold. Thus, having a "healthy" personal attitude is also important in this picture.

Rather like brushing your teeth as a child, daily exercise is a marvelous habit to get into, but one not so easily maintained when you get busy. So, the trick in fitness is

---

[10]Individuals with a history of physical problems should consult with their physician before embarking on any exercise program. If doctors say "no" to your idea, they will likely have other safe suggestions.

finding a good exercise program that fits your body and schedule.[10]

There are numerous forms of exercise available today, including mainstream hobbies like golf, swimming, hiking, and biking. In terms of spiritual exercise, however, the choices may not be so simple. Mental focus in itself is a kind of meditation. The question then becomes how beneficial that meditation is metaphysically when combined with the exercise performed. It may be that popular sports don't provide the right balance between body, mind, and soul. If that is the case, then we can look to some reborn and reinvented exercise techniques for aid.

Aerobics: The purpose for aerobics is improving the heart's efficiency and increasing the blood's oxygen capacity. Aerobic exercise helps make new blood vessels, which consequently decreases the risk of heart disease. It also helps lower blood pressure over time.

Many activities can have an aerobic quality, including dancing and walking. Jogging, running, and swimming also qualify, if they increase your heart rate and proper "cool down" periods accompany the effort.

Dance: In one of the gnostic gospels, Jesus is quoted as saying he who does not dance, does not know what happens. Maybe this idea is partially why so many cultures used dance as a way to release physical and emotional energy. Additionally, in nearly every country where you find dancing, you also find dance as a spiritual expression. African tribal cultures dance to bring about spiritual possession, whirling Dervishes dance to obtain oneness with God for divination, and the Israelites danced before the Ark of the Covenant in worship, just to name a few.

The idea of therapeutic dance among Western civilizations is credited to a German named Rudolphn Laban, who lived at the turn of the last century. When he fled to England during the war, he began working on dance movements to improve individual wellness. Today, dance aerobics remain as a tribute to his work.

Martial Arts: There are many types of martial arts from which to choose. Tai chi is a gentle, flowing art that strives to imitate nature. The movements in Tai chi restore energy while encouraging deep awareness. Ultimately, Tai chi's goal is to prevent the energy blocks that cause disease.

Aikido originated in Japan around the same time as Zen Buddhism and includes maneuvering with bladed weapons, specifically spears and swords.[11] Judo grew from jujitsu in the 1800s, also in Japan. In both cases, while the techniques were newer, the ideals behind them were very ancient. In Japan and other Eastern countries, personal control and mastery is a very honorable goal for which to strive. Physical conditioning was part of this regimen, especially for special societal classes like the Samurai.

Generally, the goal of martial arts is self-defense without weapons. However, learning other forms increases one's options and overall ability to handle diverse situations. Each has specific stances and training, most of which include breathing techniques. Trained martial artists freely allow their *chi* (force) to flow through the body.

MARTIAL ARTS AND WELLNESS by Taka[12]

Regularly practicing a martial art teaches discipline on all levels of being, and is an ongoing process for growth. If an individual practices for some time, then cannot do so, it's rather like waking up to discover you can only hear and see out of one eye or ear. The balance created through controlled regimen is disrupted, and alternatives must be found to reestablish equilibrium.

---

[11] *Karate: The Energy Connection* (New York: Delacorte Press, 1976), p. 21.
[12] Taka holds three black belts in Ju Jitsu, a black belt in Aikido, and a brown belt in Ken Jitsu after studying 22 years.

The martial arts offer an awareness of self that is always there, but not always recognized on a conscious level. This awareness, once awakened, is a powerful tool in the search for wholeness. During training you focus on all aspects of self. The goal is not just perfecting a physical form, but achieving a state of mental relaxation while enacting the art. On the spiritual level, this naturally leads to improved awareness of your place in the world and responsibilities to it. The self is connected to all other selves; that connection is inescapable, but not always understood or accepted.

Feldenkrais: Feldenkrais techniques are based on the idea that muscle tension relates directly to neurology. Specific exercises are prescribed to an individual to help reprogram patterns of the brain—basically exercising it's synapses with each movement. The exercises also stress increased awareness of posture, walking, and overall movement. Eventually a mind-body harmony is supposed to result.

Yoga: Yoga is a discipline that combines relaxation, breathing, diet, and meditation with specific physical positioning. The goal: to liberate the spirit and obtain reunion with the Divine. Certain positions are also used to help alleviate certain ailments, like a headstand that is said to cure insomnia.

While the postures of yoga are not really considered exercises, they do stretch muscles and work on balancing the spine and related systems. Controlled breathing accompanies these postures to increase personal vital force.

Walking: Early Tibetan monks took long walks to heighten altered states of awareness. And why not? It's the perfect opportunity to reconnect with the natural world and contemplate our days in privacy. Considering the fast pace our society has taken, walking may become one of the most important exercises we can do.

In choosing an exercise program that's just right for you, consider what you can really afford in the way of equipment and/or membership costs. Is the exercise sensible in terms of your climate, time constraints, location, and personal health? Don't set unsafe or unreasonable expectations. If you decide to use a facility, look for one that's conveniently located and one with flexible hours.

WELLNESS

This is an entire way of thinking. Teachers of wellness stress our lifestyle and mindset as being the key to health. Here, one maintains fitness through a stable diet, regular exercise, by changing behavior patterns, and making wise personal choices, rather than waiting until sickness occurs.

Wellness is not something that happens overnight. It is a learning process motivated by a strong personal desire to be truly whole in body and spirit. In terms of successful exercise, wellness experts recommend working with a group, exercising to music, keeping a progress chart, and getting people you know to encourage your efforts.

Before beginning a workout, one should stretch, as this reduces muscle strain and prepares the body for activity. Aerobics, isotonics to improve strength and endurance, flexion routines, and balancing exercises are all recommended in this regimen. Specific, common exercises from this list include cycling, jumping rope, and swimming.

In terms of diet, everything discussed in the section on "Food" in this chapter applies. Additionally, wellness managers encourage their students to stop "eating their words" and "swallowing one's pride." Believe it or not, this can lead to many different maladies including ulcers and obesity! Why? Because such actions force down emotions and personal vision, making the individual uncomfortable and ill at ease.

Last, but not least, wellness advisors remind us that rest and relaxation are important parts of the health equation too. All work and no play not only makes "Jack a dull boy," but also subjects "Jack" to any number of illnesses that could have been avoided by a decent night's sleep. Everything we want to accomplish mundanely and spiritually will be achieved far better with a rested, nourished body. So, be well!

12

Homeopathy:
Aroma, Flower, and Sound Therapy

*Practitioners of all disciplines must first and foremost
acquire an understanding of natural law and
medicine which regards man in a holistic framework.*
—Dr. Wallace F. MacNaughton

HOLISTIC ATTITUDES HAVE BEEN WITH HUMAN-
kind for a very long time, evidencing themselves regularly
in "occult" techniques. Even Socrates said, "There is no illness of the body apart from the mind." Thus, treating the
mind and body as a whole is the essence of holistic therapy.

While there are many severe critics of alternative medicine, most of whom regard holistics as a pseudoscience, the
history and regularity of effectiveness of the techniques
cannot be dismissed. Homeopathy was founded in the
1800s by Samuel Hahnemann, a German physician. Dr.
Hahnemann assembled hundreds of homeopathic medica-
tions from plants, animals, and minerals through conscien-
tious research. Later, his concepts traveled with immigrants
to the United States where they found a welcome home. By
1900, there were 22 homeopathic schools and over 100 hospitals devoted to this form of treatment.[1] Homeopathy also
gained some rather notable proponents, including Mother
Theresa and Queen Elizabeth II.

---

[1]Time-Life Books, eds., *Powers of Healing,* (Alexandria, VA: Time-Life
Books, 1989), p. 120.

The key to homeopathy is the "law of similars," which we see readily in things like smallpox vaccines. Hippocrates understood this all too well when he said, "Through the application of the like, it [disease] is cured."[2] A secondary key for homeopathy is the belief that only a small catalyst is necessary to stimulate the body's healing mechanism.

Experiments performed by Dr. Jaques Benveniste in the 1980s seem to bear out the truth of this second idea by showing a biological response to one specific, highly diluted antibody. While his experiments have been refuted by some, they have never been totally discredited. Dr. Benveniste believes that diluted substances still bear a chemical imprint, or memory, which is passed on to the body by internalization. That memory then becomes a building block for wholeness by stimulating the cells toward their normal, healthy condition.

Overall, a homeopath's job is one of careful observation. Everything about a patient must be noted to decipher the best, most effective route to wellness. Returning to the concept of holistics, the condition of the patient's body, mind, and spirit are all accounted for before any prescriptions are made. A homeopath is also a teacher. As they review a patient's condition and begin treatment, homeopaths provide information on movement, diet, environment, the psyche, body chemistry, and other factors that may hinder (or help) wellness. This educates the patient about universal relationships as they pertain specifically to that individual. In the process, other specialists may be recommended, especially in chronic cases.

Homeopathic treatments are about 60 percent botanically based. The remainder comes from minerals, animal products, or extremely diluted disease extracts. Herbalists will be quick to point out, however, that, while homeopathy uses botanical essences, it is not a field of herbalism, since

---

[2]George Vithoulkas, *The Science of Homeopathy* (Athens: Athenian School of Homeopathic Medicine, 1978), p. 113.

the two systems approach their final treatment in vastly different ways.

During homeopathic treatments (which may occur singly or in a series), it is not uncommon to have external manifestations of an illness get temporarily worse. Ultimately, the human body wants to expel sickness—to move it outward. Consequently, internal problems can get better while other side effects of treatment, like hives may appear externally. Also, the upper body tends to improve before the lower, but this is only a generality not a hard and fast rule.[3]

Additionally, some things seem to have a negative or nullifying effect on homeopathic treatments, including camphor, menthols, salts, certain cosmetics, soaps, and even common aspirin. Because of this, it is essential that a patient receive full instructions from their homeopath regarding "dos" and "don'ts." Any patient undergoing homeopathic treatment should always make other physicians (like dentists) aware of this so two different approaches to medicine don't collide with adverse results.

Some people like to try "over the counter" homeopathic cures themselves for common ailments. Health-food stores and cooperatives sometimes sell what are considered homeopathic "first aid" kits. These kits usually include some aconite for colds and fever, wild hops for an ill temperament, chamomile for insomnia, and rue for bruises and headaches, as well as other items. Take care, however, in choosing a homeopathic kit. I do not recommend getting it from any unlicensed company or individual, as some homeopathic cures utilize substances that are highly dangerous in inexperienced hands. Additionally, it is prudent to obtain some sound books on homeopathy before trying anything. One title to consider is *Everybody's Guide to Homeo-*

---

[3]The rules about how homeopathic cures evidence themselves originated with Constantine Hering, a German immigrant of the 1830s. Hering's hand was saved from amputation by homeopathy, making him a steadfast convert. He personally founded three homeopathic schools.

pathic Medicine by Dana Ullmann, available through J. P. Tarcher (1984).

Homeopathy is aimed toward people who desire a greater understanding of themselves and their environment. It is designed to aid the evolution toward spiritual, physical, and emotional wholeness by exploring the deeper causes of dis-ease. For further information, call or write:

Institute for Classical
  Homeopathy
1336 Oak Ave.
St. Helena, CA 94574
Phone: 415-248-1632

National Center for
  Homeopathy
801 N. Fairfax #306
Alexandria, VA 22314
Phone: 703-548-7790

HERBALISM

Herbalism has its roots deep in antiquity. The interest in natural medicine and the use of nonchemical health aids has grown steadily over the last century, delayed only briefly by popular medicalization at the turn of the century. Even at that juncture, however, books such as the *Family Botanic Guide* by William Fox (1907) was in its 18th edition! This type of guide, common during the Victorian era, seems to typify what we now see, in that they contain constant references to older texts of great healers such as Culpepper, Galen, Paracelsus, and Hippocrates.

Herbalism has been used effectively by wives, warriors, charlatans, doctors, and dreamers of all eras, probably because it was readily accessible. Thus healthful, helpful herbs find their way into everything, including:

Teas and infusions	Creams and oils
Poultices, plasters, and compresses	Powders
Tinctures	Syrups
Washes and baths	Inhalants
Aromatics (perfume, potpourri)	Cookery

The oldest written records on this art were discovered in Egypt, China, and India. The Chinese penned herbal curatives as early as 3737 B.C. Egyptian papyri dated 2,000 B.C. refer to even older documents. In India, herbalism was called Ayurveda around 1,000 B.C., but this was only the beginning.

Hippocrates directed medicine toward a science and recommended many herbal prescriptions in 3 B.C., with two books on this subject. Pliny the Elder penned 37 books of *Natural History* in the first century, incorporating many natural remedies and tidbits of folk medicine. Galen and Dioscorides arrived on the scene during the Greco-Roman period, both writing antidotes and recipes and collecting herbal information for future herbalists to ponder.

Yet, of all periods in history, the one richest in herbal remnants is the Middle Ages. Quite properly known as the Age of Herbals, the Middle Ages abounds in beautiful manuscripts that were carefully copied by monks documenting every aspect of the herbal arts, from growing and harvesting to actual application. Mixed liberally into these writings were remnants of earlier ideas on sympathy and the divine signature in nature that allowed healers to know what plants to use for what ailments—for example, using a yellow-colored flower as part of a cure for jaundice.

Alongside more medically based curatives, the manuscripts also show herbs being used for emotional and mundane trauma. Parsley was taken to prevent drunkenness, anise banished nightmares, basil relieved hatred, and laurel invoked the gift of prophesy. Some of these ideas were adopted from Arabic traders, looking to improve the price of their wares. Others, however, came from a more ancient and venerable source: the oral tradition of cunning folk, mothers, and healers.

Thankfully, the Church was unable to completely banish these traditional applications or their subtler holistic, metaphysical message. This is the message that New Age herbalists heed, then add an awareness of toxicity and other factors of which the ancients were unaware. In this manner, the best of the old and new meet in a marvelous marriage to create improved wellness for all.

One common misconception about herbalism that needs clarifying at this juncture is that this art only pertains to "herbs." This is not at all true. Much of what has been categorized historically and in modern times about herbalism includes flowers, roots, trees, fruits, and vegetables, as well as spices. In this respect, I regard herbalism as a broad ranging dietary supplement that considers nature's warehouse as a medicine cabinet, waiting to be opened.

Willow bark, for example, makes an incredibly effective aspirin alternative, and dandelions are a good tonic, their juice being an excellent skin conditioner! You will find neither of these on a supermarket shelf. Even so, modern science has validated these applications, which certainly ease both discomfort and one's budget!

Drawbacks

Today, herbal correspondences for health and spirituality can readily be found in New Age books, thanks to dedicated scribes of old. With legalities being very complex, however, someone who is a practicing herbalist must either get state or local licensing, or be very careful about how and when they share any type of "advice." Personally, I usually keep my preparations within the realm of what I call "pleasure herbalism," including creams, scented oils, incense, and soap. Even with items as simple as these, I still have to take great care to check about people's allergies.

Another difficulty in herbalism is one that I rarely read about in books: varying environments. Growing seasons do not produce the exact same potencies in essential oils, vitamins, and the other beneficial qualities of an herb. Changes in soil, sunlight, rain, and other environmentally caused conditions can also alter these qualities. As a result, herbalism is never an exact art; yet it is one that must be measured and tested carefully, using the herbalists' rede: "If one can cure, two can kill."

Finally, in recent years the AMA has begun to observe and monitor the herbal market closely, threatening to take even benign items like chamomile out of the public sector. This, indeed, would be a terrible loss. I agree that herbal businesses need regulation to ensure that "organics" are truly organic, and that one green leafy thing isn't packaged as another. Nonetheless, after all the progress toward holistic approaches we've seen of late, removing many herbal preparations from the market would seem a giant step backward. This means herbalists, and those who support them, will have to be very active politically to keep their art from being extinguished by red tape.

Advantages

With that said, there are many things about herbalism that I love and teach readily. Most of the herbs in your own pantry can be used for maintaining the body, improving the mind, and calming the spirit. A list of these applications follows later in this chapter.

Since culinary herbs are also some of the safest in generally accepted cooking quantities, they are also the easiest ones to learn and apply to help ease common maladies. For example, if everyone has been getting colds lately, make a soup that includes fresh garlic, nettle, sage, and thyme. These items often go into soup anyway, so they won't leave an odd flavor behind. Upon internalization, their natural magic begins!

At no time should this approach be considered a replacement for modern medicine. If symptoms persist, see your doctor. Prudence does not equate to a lack of faith; it is wisdom in action!

MOM'S TEA by Marian

Everyone, including 30-year old friends, call me "Mom." It seems to be a label that suits, as I always seem to fit that description in one form or another. In recent years, these people have frequently come to me, when feeling ill with a cold or flu, for some of my tea. While inevitably they turn up their nose and make terrible faces upon drinking it, every year they come back for another dose! Why? Because it works.

Rosehips provide Vitamin C, orange and lemon rind help cut phlegm, chamomile and mint settle the stomach and nerves, eucalyptus breaks up congestion, and a bit of ginger increases circulation and energy. Yes, it tastes terrible. I jokingly say that it has to taste that way—like any good medicine—or it wouldn't be effective!

All these ingredients are easily accessible through cooperatives and other places that sell bulk herbs. I always tell those who ask for teas (or any preparation) that the recipe is based on several sources, but that results aren't guaranteed. Likewise, I'm careful about telling them the ingredients to avoid allergic reactions, and I never recommend any teas to pregnant women that aren't professionally prepared and certified as organic.[4] I do not feel that such precautions relinquish the power of herbal arts to dogma and nitpicking. These are sensible safeguards for responsible people, who likewise wish to help their friends and family naturally.

HERBS AND THEIR USES

Below I have provided a very abbreviated list of some of the more common herbs and their healthful applications. As seen in sections of this book on aromatherapy and Bach's

---

[4]Many herbs and the pesticides used in growing them can inadvertently cause miscarriage. Always consult a professional herbalist and your physician when choosing herbal supplements during pregnancy.

remedies, this list is truly only the tip of the proverbial iceberg. It does not begin to share metaphysical correspondences that can likewise aid the spirit, and can only provide a cursory look at emotional uses. This is a study worthy of tomes, so, as you read, please bear in mind that one section of a book cannot adequately cover the herbal arts. If you're interested in this field, I highly recommend reading authors like Scott Cunningham (metaphysical), Jude Williams (physical, practical), Louise Riotte (practical, historical, gardening), and Rev. Paul Beyerl (religious, healthful).

Aloe: Burn ointment and skin conditioner.

Anise: Digestive aid, decreases flatulence, eases cough and, as a tea, is said to avert nightmares.

Basil: Dispelling cramps, loosening constipation, calming anxiety or stress.

Bay: Increased courage and strength. Externally a rub for sore joints. Internally applied for soothing the stomach.

Birch: An excellent gargle. In teas used for headache and fever, in poultice form, to soothe wounds of a minor nature.

Burdock: A blood purifier and laxative. The root is good for skin conditions. Symbolically, an emblem of humble fortunes. Considered by some cultures as a vegetable.

Catnip: Digestive and sleep aid.

Chamomile: Calming nerves, headaches, or a restless tummy. In oil/lotion form, a good anti-inflammatory.

Chive: Dispels negativity. Vapors cleanse sinuses. In larger quantities, akin to onion for aiding blood pressure.

Dandelion: Root used for liver troubles. Plant itself builds the blood, averting anemia. Increases appetite. Spiritually, the flower of ancient oracles.

Dill: Protective herb, especially against magic. Increases mother's milk, decreases colic and flatulence.

Fennel: Dietary aid, increases vigor, improves digestion. Mild stimulant.

Garlic: Kills germs, especially yeasts like those present in foot fungus. Treatment for respiratory ailments and high blood pressure.

Ginger: Eases indigestion, good breath freshener and energy enhancer. Promotes circulation.

Hops: Mild sedative.

Onion: Good expectorant, diuretic, and antiseptic. Decreases asthma, blood pressure, headaches, and congestion.

Peppermint: Calming chills, stomach upset, or headache.

Rose: In an infusion, good for colds, due to high vitamin C content. Syrup recommended for throat infections.

Sage: In an infusion, applied to colds, dizziness, nausea, and poor digestion. Also good as a gargle and overall rinse for the gums and mouth.

Thyme: Antiseptic, carminative, and antispasmodic qualities. Treatment for bronchial problems, stomach and intestinal discomfort.

13

Massage, Reflexology, and Therapeutic Touch

The hands speak themselves.
—Quintilian

TOUCH IS IMPORTANT TO ALL HANDS-ON HEALERS. In this chapter we shall look at massage, reflexology, and what we call therapeutic touch because all of these techniques are important for the healing process.

MASSAGE

Massage moved into the modern world without difficulty. It is comforting, alleviates aches, and soothes the stress from our busy routines. The term "massage" comes from the Greek *masso*, meaning "I knead." The technique has ancient roots and some very famous proponents, including Hippocrates, who left directions for massage in his writings for other healers to follow.

A Greek physician named Asclepiades relied exclusively on massage to restore nutritive fluids in the body to a healthy state. Caesar used massage to offset the effects of epilepsy. Pliny, a Roman scholar, used it to aid his personal asthma. And a 2,000-year-old alabaster relief currently on display at the Pergamon Museum of Berlin depicts the massage of an Assyrian leader.

For a while during the early Middle Ages, massage fell into disuse, possibly due to the Church's disapproval. It was not until the late 1500s that French physicians and surgeons started reexploring manipulative techniques. Three hundred years later, massage became recognized in Europe as a beneficial technique, particularly to aid athletes. Germany, Austria, and France became leaders in this area, including physical therapy, until the 1920s when massage finally gained interest in the United States. Even then, it was not until the 1980s that massage therapy was portrayed as a reputable occupation, primarily due to the holistic movement.

There are quite literally dozens of massage methods that I discovered during research, including some geared specifically to animals or children. A few that are worthy of note are: Bindegewebsmassage, which comes from Germany, and uses skin stimulation to affect other areas of the body; Esalen-style massage, which originated in the 1960s and is more sensual, intuitive, and nurturing than clinical; the Rosen method, also from Germany, which utilizes touch, bodywork, and communication to decrease pain and improve emotional awareness; and Thai massage, which developed around the second century B.C., combining traditional Chinese methods and meridians with yoga and aspects of Hindu philosophy. This last technique is often familial, its secrets passed from parent to child.

Whatever the approach, massage therapy is very effective in treating pain, decreasing stress, and improving circulation. Good practitioners begin slowly and cautiously until they learn the intricacies of the body they are treating. Some may combine their work with subliminal tapes, instrumental music, gentle talk, and other methods to make the patient more comfortable.

While general massage can be learned by just about anyone, a massage therapist must be licensed. For someone less trained, the best advice is to be careful. Ask a person about any injuries they've incurred, or how they like their backrubs in terms of pressure. This will keep you from inadvertently causing pain instead of peacefulness.

Useful addresses:

Body Mind & Spirit
917-2 N. Main St.
Toms River, NJ 08753
Phone: 908-349-7153

Institute for Therapeutic
    Massage
Phone: 973-839-6131

Rosen Center West
Box 344
Sante Fe, NM 87504
Phone: 510-845-6606
1-800-893-2622 (referrals)

Esalen Institute
Highway 1
Big Sur, CA 93920
Phone: 408-667-3000

Lomilomi
1779 E. Main St.
Ventura, CA 93001
Phone: 800-514-0147

REFLEXOLOGY

Reflexology employs pressure points on the feet or hands, in combination with massage, to obtain results similar to those which acupressure gives. Each point or zone corresponds to major organs and areas of the body. The concept behind reflexology may be quite old, considering that Egyptian, Chinese, and Indian illustrations and texts all have instances of foot massage. While a reflexologist will quickly point out that this technique is not strictly "massage," it seems the ancients were aware that some type of pressure to the feet was beneficial.

Like other homeopathic approaches, Reflexology is a synergistic art. Each foot contains over 7,000 nerve endings that connect to other parts of the body.[1] This makes the feet an ideal starting point for relaxation and blockage release. Additionally, it allows the practitioner to treat injuries that might not normally be accessible to other therapies, like broken bones. By working on the corresponding spot on the foot, a reflexologist can provide pain relief without ever touching the inflicted spot.

Many reflexologists report that this work takes approximately half the time when combined with the principles of massage therapy, which is why they are both included in this chapter. For patients who are uncomfortable with, or unaccustomed to, touch, reflexology offers one means for a therapist to begin opening that door so other therapies can follow if needed. Except for the overtly ticklish, the feet and hands are neutral zones, perceived as safe by most people.

Reflexology is not considered an exact science, as the points that affect each individual will vary. Nonetheless, certain correlations exist. There is a strong connection between the arms, legs, and shoulders and the hands and feet because of their proximity.

Overall, reflexology takes about 200 hours of solid classroom and field experience to learn proficiently. Not all programs are alike, however, and any potential student should check out any instructor or program under consideration thoroughly. For more information contact:

NYS Reflexology Assoc.
Phone: 716-693-3068

International Institute of
  Reflexology
Box 12642
St. Petersburg, FL 33733-2642

---

[1] *Massage Magazine*, Carolyn K. Long, "Reflexology," Issue 59, p. 27.

THERAPEUTIC TOUCH

In considering therapeutic touch and its benefits, remember that the concept of "laying on of hands" is very old, having a place in both religion and health. Even Stone Age artists depicted healing hands hard at work, and a great Roman physician, Galen, used massage as a healing method in the second century A.D. The New Testament also repeatedly discusses the hand as a channel for divine energy. This indicates that, while people at early historical junctures may not have totally understood the importance of touch, they were intuitively aware of its comforting effects.

As time wore on, the belief in the efficacy of touch remained firm. In the Middle Ages, the touch of a King could help heal the sick. During the 1600s a man by the name of Valentine Greatrakes traveled throughout London performing miracles by the laying on of hands. Contemporary evangelicals and New Agers alike still use this approach. So the question becomes: why is touch so important and how does it affect our psyches?

Skin represents the largest organ of the human body, filled with nerve cells that transmit messages to the mind. Thus, when the skin receives comfort or has an experience, so does the brain, which then sends that message to the rest of the body. In a very real sense, this means our bodies have memories locked away in skin cells, muscles, and connective tissues.

Consider for a moment some modern phrases. We call people "soft touches," discuss "rubbing someone the wrong way," or how someone "gets under our skin"! When something is uncertain, it's "touch and go." If someone is too harsh or too sensitive, they're "heavy handed" or "thin skinned," respectively. All of this points to the importance of touch and its effect on human awareness, interactions, and, inevitably, wellness. Add to this the fact that touching the skin is also one way to come into direct contact with the most intimate portion of a person's aura and you have a very potent tool. Touch transmits energy directly into the patient's aura for the most beneficial and least disruptive results.

With this foundational information in mind, Dr. Dolores Kreiger at New York University began studying and detailing the effects of therapeutic touch. At first, Ms. Kreiger (who was then an RN) remained skeptical, becoming an outside observer to others who used the laying on of hands to heal the sick. Over time and with observation, however, she was so impressed by what she saw, that her doctoral thesis researched this healing process. Once its effects were documented, Dr. Kreiger provided instructions to help other healers learn this technique. First, healers must be at peace with themselves and learn to separate their feelings and problems from those of the patient. Secondly, healers need to focus, firmly setting aside the self and directing their whole attention to the person in need. Next, they should study the patient's energy fields, making a mental note of everything—this is the assessment period. Any obstructed energy must be freed (called "unruffling the field"). Then, healers direct energy to help the patient return to symmetry. Finally, but most importantly, healers have to know when to stop, which is indicated by the lack of continued input or cues from the aura.

Most people who work with therapeutic touch also perform auric cleansing and balancing in the process, as sensing blocked or imbalanced energy requires an intimate awareness of the aura. (For more information on these two techniques, return to Part II, chapter 3.) Because of this focus on physical and emotional energy fields, therapeutic touch has proven itself to be very helpful for people experiencing chronic pain, or in comforting terminally ill patients (pain relievers, emotional care-givers, and, potentially, physical manifestors). It is also useful in working with young children and animals, both of whom are very open to auric input. In these instances, however, treatment should be applied for shorter periods.

Glorious Relief

In 1988 I was in a head-on collision wherein a vertebrae between my shoulder blades was fractured and compressed. At the same time, all the ligaments down both sides of my spine tore, my right knee hit the dashboard, and my hips smashed into the steering wheel. Laying on the backboard in the hospital was horribly frightening. After all, my son was only 2. I had no idea how I would cope.

After coming home in a backbrace, and being in continuous pain for many weeks, I was encouraged by a friend to take a trip to see some people he knew. One of them was very skilled in therapeutic touch. The healer gently encouraged me to give it a fair chance at least—and since the medication wasn't helping I was open to just about any possibility that could provide relief.

I didn't realize until well into this first session that therapeutic touch has a mesmerizing effect. The healer's soft voice, music, and gentle movements seem to guide the body and mind naturally into relaxed, nearly visionary states. Slowly, as the therapist worked, everything outside seemed to disappear. Nothing existed but the rhythm of my heart—there was no pain, no time, no concrete world to hold me down. I felt as if I were floating in another realm. It was an incredibly liberating experience.

Afterward, when I got off the work table, my shock must have been obvious. It was the first time since my accident that I could move without wincing! While the effect was temporary, I got a full night's sleep—the first since my injury; that alone was a tremendous gift. My sleepless nights had left me very frazzled, feeling helpless, and slowly slipping into depression. The rest snapped me out of that cycle, and knowing there was a treatment that could ease the pain provided hope and motivation.

Since that time I have learned to use therapeutic touch to help others. Every time I begin to work on someone at home, I'm amazed and amused by children and animals insisting on being in the room. Cats roll around near the patient as if the energy were catnip, and the children just watch curiously, as if absorbing information.

Therapeutic touch does require a certain empathy with the patient's problems. As is the case with many of the intimate types of healing discussed in this chapter, this creates one hazard. Healers must take extra care not to accept sickness into themselves during therapy. If they lose their center point while they're working, it can open the door to such an occurrence.[2] So, healers must act only as intermediaries between sickness and health, basically funneling any negative energy out of themselves and into the earth.[3]

The most remarkable thing about therapeutic touch is its unadorned, pragmatic ideology. Dr. Krieger claims no miracles. Studies performed by Dr. Krieger and others, however, have shown that therapeutic touch affects blood composition and brain waves, as well as encouraging the relaxation response in patients, which is perhaps the most important aspect of this technique.

Dr. Krieger believes that everyone can develop healing hands with time and practice. She has personally taught over 20,000 people therapeutic touch and has been an integral driving force in getting this method accepted into many hospital programs.[4] In her own words: "I am thoroughly convinced that the ability to use Therapeutic Touch

---

[2]Dolores Krieger, *The Therapeutic Touch* (New York: Fireside, 1979), p. 41.
[3]Please take care that you don't accidentally splash pets or plants with residual dis-ease. One good option here is to have a bowl of wash water or rich soil in which to immerse your hands periodically.
[4]Time-Life Editors, *Powers of Healing* (Alexandria, VA: Time-Life Books, 1989), p. 107.

is a natural potential in man which can be actualized under the appropriate conditions."[5]

Part of the reason this technique is easy for most people to learn is the individualization that Dr. Kreiger stresses. Repeatedly in her work, she reminds us that healers must find their own personal cues to guide their hand movements and everything else done to open a channel and direct energy. She also emphasizes that intention and motivation are just as important as technique in being successful. For more information on therapeutic touch, write:

Therapeutic Touch
  Massage Clinic
607 Main #1020
Houston, TX 77030
Phone: 713-795-5885

In Touch Bodywork
301 N. Water St.
Milwaukee, WI 53202
Phone: 404-289-9164

National Certification Board
  for Therapeutic Massage and Bodywork
8201 Greensboro Dr. #300
McLean, VA 22102
Phone: 1-800-296-0664

---

[5]Dolores Krieger, *Therapeutic Touch*, from the preface.

14

Meditation
(Past-Life Regression and Rebirthing)

And let us all to meditation.
—Shakespeare

OF ALL ALTERNATIVE HEALING TECHNIQUES TO reach the public, meditation and visualization have been among the most widely accepted. Possibly this is because they require no specific belief system to be effective. Nearly all physicians readily agree that a patient's state of mind is just as important as medication, possibly more so. For the purpose of this book, however, we will examine meditation and visualization solely in New Age terms and in various applied spiritual settings.

THE CONTEMPLATIVE PATH

Overall, meditation is one technique that we all can work into our daily routine successfully. It helps reduce stress, improves the workings of the immune system, decreases chronic pain, normalizes blood pressure, and generally helps keep things on an even keel.[1] In fact, nearly every healer interviewed for this book uses meditation in some form to aid themselves or their patients.

Meditation is a tool taught to people to help increase spiritual, mental, and/or physical awareness. Exactly what happens during that process depends on the meditation's objective and the procedure itself. Specifically, someone desiring improved creative flow approaches the meditative process differently than a healer or someone who needs healing.

Additionally, different religious systems treat meditation from distinctly unique vantage points. Some use it to create the proper state of mind for ritual, while others adapt it as a means of focusing energy. Some use meditation as a vehicle for drawing sacred power; others use it to cleanse themselves of impurity. Taoists, for example, meditate to banish unwanted thoughts and bring an inner stillness.[2] Ayurvedic philosophers employ meditation for mental hygiene wherein the mind sits quietly in an expanded state.[3]

Meditative principles go back to at least 200 B.C., mostly as a religious expression. Today, however, psychologists and metaphysicians recognize that meditation can have many other potentially positive applications including relieving the anxiety and negative thought patterns of daily life. Transcendental meditation, for example,

---

[1.] See Dr. Herbert Benson *The Relaxation Response* (New York: Avon, 1976. The findings of Dr. Benson were confirmed by other published studies on the effects of meditation and yoga, specifically *Love, Medicine & Miracles* by Bernie Siegel (New York: HarperCollins, 1990), pp. 150–153.

[2]Denny Sargent, *Global Ritualism* (St. Paul, MN: Llewellyn Publications, 1994), p. 14. This is an excellent book of comparative worldwide religion/ritual, complete with photographs.

[3]Time-Life Editors, *Powers of Healing* (Alexandria, VA: Time-Life Books, 1989), p. 66.

uses calm visions or soothing phrases as a focus for de-creasing tension.

Ultimately, the purpose of meditation in healing is fourfold. First, it puts both healer and patient in receptive states of mind through which wholesome energy can flow freely. Secondly, it helps relax nervous patients who feel silly, uncertain, or vulnerable. Third, by meditating to-gether, both healer and patient harmonize their energies, making the healer's job much easier. Last, but not least, it provides a more detached perspective that allows both par-ties to tackle the illness objectively.

MEDITATIVE AIDS

One may meditate without visualization, since meditation is basically a deeply thoughtful state, akin to prayer. Yet, most people find that imagery helps them focus on a goal. Addi-tionally, other elements can be added to meditations to make them more effective and geared toward a specific purpose. Included in this list are affirmations, mantras, chanting, and breathing.

Breathing: Breathing helps develop your concentration. Healers use breath to help convey positive energy toward their patients as well as a cleansing mechanism for them-selves. Individuals using meditation for healing also use paced breathing as a way to center their attention on the matter at hand, and thereby open their spiritual awareness.

For relaxation, the pattern breathing most frequently takes is that of deep, cyclical inhalation through the nose, and exhalation through the mouth. If you try this yourself three times slowly, you will immediately notice that your shoulders relax a bit, and you can almost sense your center of gravity (near the navel). The calming, centering effect of this pattern is exactly why it's so popular among healers.

Once someone has established a meditative state, they may change their focus away from breathing to the heartbeat, especially for health matters. Blood carries life-affirming oxygen to the body. By paying attention to that center, the healer and patient can convey white-light energy through a natural, established physical current, giving a whole new meaning to the modern phrase: "Go with the flow!"

Autogenics and Hypnosis: This particular technique was developed in the 1920s by Johannes Schultz, a German psychiatrist. Basically, autogenics uses specific exercises to help induce meditative or hypnotic states. These activities include allowing one's limbs to feel heavy and warm, calming the heartbeat, a focus on breathing, and cooling the forehead.

Once these simple methods are mastered, people can learn how to aid their own recuperative processes. Only minor changes occur from person to person, depending on the problem. For example, a person with a sore arm would probably not be instructed to sense that area as "warm," because heat can emphasize pain.

It is undeniable that autogenics resembles hypnosis, except that, ultimately, autogenics can be administered by the individual. Conversely, in hypnotism, the healer guides the patient through word and visualization toward a specific goal that may be subliminally or consciously implanted during the session. Both approaches use the receptive state of the patient as a vehicle for improved wellness. While self-hypnosis is possible for some people, many find that having a guide helps. This allows patients to direct their attention away from the process and put more focus on the predominant goal.

Affirmation: Language is powerful and transformational. In *Words of Power* by Brian and Esther Crowley, we read, "the use of sound for specific purposes is universal and historical."[4] During the Middle Ages, jongleurs used language to influence the emotions of their listeners. In the Book of Genesis, God created the world by expressing words of command.

Thus, an affirmation is just one way of tapping the latent energy in our own speech. Affirmations equate to short, positive, repeated phrases, stated throughout meditation to emphasize specific energies. By speaking and listening during moments of total inner peacefulness, we draw that specific spoken vibration into ourselves. Functional examples for self-healing include "I am healthy," "I am whole," and "I accept peace and inner harmony." To change this for someone administering affirmations as part of the healing process, simply substitute "you" for "I."

Mantra: Mantras also focus on wordpower for wellness. A mantra utilizes words or syllables whose rhythm and sound produce an altered state of consciousness.[5] The Tibetan AUM is perhaps the most widely known example. Some people choose to follow a set mantra which comes from a specific tradition, while others discover a personal mantra during their meditations.

The best example I have for this is personal. Many years ago, while in a deeply meditative state, words began filling my mind. It was a seven-syllable sentence which repeated itself until I had it memorized. Not knowing or understanding why I had received what seemed like "babble," the only thing I could equate this to was the phenomenon of speaking in tongues—the indwelling of the Holy Spirit experienced by some Christian sects.

---

[4]Brian & Esther Crowley, *Words of Power* (St. Paul, MN: Llewellyn Publications, 1991), p. 5.
[5]Diane Mariechild, *Mother Wit* (Freedom, CA: Crossing Press, 1988) p. 24.

Finally, I got up the nerve to ask someone more experienced if my conclusion was correct. Much to my surprise, they said that a mantra could be similar to tongues, only of a more personal nature (instead of a communal message). They went on to explain that mantras may or may not incorporate words from a known language. In my case, each word was fairly close to a discernable term from various countries. As I became more familiar with New Age techniques, I discovered that these countries were places I'd lived in past lives!

While this specific experience had little to do with healing, except to make me feel less crazy about my faith, it helps illustrate the foundational matrix of mantras. A mantra reaffirms your spiritual life and path. It expresses your vibration in the orchestra of the universe. Repeating mantras brings a patient or healer into symmetry with sacred energy.

Biofeedback: The principles of biofeedback teach individuals to recognize the relationship between mind and body, and how to control specific bodily functions. I've had the opportunity to experience this method firsthand, and it's quite interesting.

To begin with, the patient is hooked up to a brain-wave monitor, then asked to relax. As the patient relaxes, the sounds emitted from the monitor become more pleasant, basically rewarding the effort. Using the sound as a guide, people learn to hone in on specific mental vibrations appropriate to their physical goals.

I had approached biofeedback as an experiment to see what level of meditation I could achieve under rather chaotic circumstances. After about twenty minutes of settling in, the majority of the readings were on the theta level (creative and meditative), with some alpha mingling in (relaxation)—basically, a good sign.

The only problem was that the person administering the test got excited enough when a delta wave showed up (this usually comes during sleep, but can also indicate inspiring ideas) to shout. That effectively ended the experiment and left me with a terrific headache for coming out too quickly! All in all, however, I would have to say this was a positive experience. I think it could be most helpful in teaching workaholics how to relax!

Visualization: Visualization relies on the amazing powers of the mind as its foundation. If you watch young children during a sad movie, you will realize that they cannot define the difference between what is imagined and what is real. Successful visualization depends on our ability to tap that particular portion of our mind, at any age, that is still childlike in its acceptance of "truth." The idea is to fool the body into thinking that our mental images are real physical experiences.

Beyond this, visualization allows patients to become more intimately involved in their own well-being. Consequently, patients experience an increased feeling of control, instead of the sickness ruling their every action. This, in itself, is an important mental advantage that works toward health. Repeatedly seeing cancerous cells overcome by healthy ones, for example, inspires hope, which motivates specific physical responses that eventually help renew the patient.

VISUALIZATION by Arawn Machia[6]

A lot of people have problems with visualization. Somehow they equate it with youthful flights of fancy for which they got reprimanded. So, the first step in visualization therapy is letting people know it's "ok" to dream and use their imagination. Relaxation

---

[6]See also Part II, chapter 3, "Auric Cleansing and Balancing." Used by permission.

methods like breathing can help this process along by getting the patient into a mental space that encourages more freedom.

Once you're beyond that barrier, visualization may take two directions. The first is guiding the patient from beginning to end. The second is taking the visualization to a point, then allowing the patient to develop the visualization themselves. Each has its benefits.

There is an old aphorism that says: "Seeing is believing." Essentially this is the basis for all visualization exercises. If one can see wellness, they can be well. The potential is there simply waiting for something to set the process in motion. Visualization can not only provide that impetus initially, but later provides positive imagery to keep wellness as an evolving, kinetic power in the patient's mind.

Visualization is productive in both groups and individuals, making it tremendously flexible to a diversity of needs. Among groups, it is easiest to work with archetypal forms to which the whole group can relate. For individuals, the images need to make sense in their reality. As a case in point, Christians will get a far better mental image of the Holy Spirit, than they would of the New Age term "White Light."

In either instance, a healer should lay good groundwork before visualization begins. Jumping in and expecting people to see complex scenes is unrealistic and unproductive. Visualization needs to be goal-oriented from start to finish, wherein the healer's presence comforts the patient, never abandoning them to images that can be unnerving.

Another benefit to visualization is for healers themselves to use. Visualizing your healing method (and perfecting it in the visualization) becomes like a dress rehearsal that builds confidence and often lends astounding insight. Also, visualization helps offset energy drains when needs arise unexpectedly. In this instance, try seeing yourself immersed in one of the four elements (earth, air, fire, water) to which you most strongly respond. Allow this to feed your inner well until you can meet your tasks refreshed. This is only a temporary solution that should not replace self-care. A healer's body is a temple to care for elegantly.

Sample Guided Meditation/Visualization for Overcoming a Cold

The speaker throughout this example is the healer, who gently guides the patient to a deeply relaxed state. Once healers feel the patient is ready, they provide descriptive imagery for overcoming the physical, emotional, or spiritual problem:

Begin by taking three deep breaths, slowly, in through your nose and out through your mouth **[pause and observe]**.

Good **[healer always reaffirms when patient is approaching the process correctly]**. Now, one more time, even more slowly. As you exhale feel your tensions flowing away from you **[pause]**.

Relax, rest . . . there is no need to hurry or rush now. You are safe, peaceful, and totally at ease. Relax your forehead . . . let it become smooth, carefree . . . relax your face . . . your neck . . . your shoulders **[pause]**. As you relax your arms and hands, they start to feel heavy . . . then your thighs . . . heavy and deeply relaxed . . . calves . . . deeply relaxed . . . feet . . . deeply relaxed **[healer pauses here to assess the patient's body language. If necessary the healer will continue the relaxation, repeating any areas that still appear tense]**.

Excellent. You are now totally relaxed and comfortable. Keep breathing in through your nose and out through your mouth. Listen to that breath, let it connect with itself . . . let it flow, bringing oxygen to your body **[pause]**. When you feel ready, I want you to visualize yourself in someplace that is totally peaceful . . . a place where you are always happy and safe **[pause until the patient's face**

smiles naturally]. It is a beautiful sunny day, with a light, comfortable breeze.

Find someplace comfortable to sit down or lie down in the sunlight. Sense the warmth of the sun on your skin . . . feel that warmth filling every cell with refreshed energy **[pause]**. Imagine that the Sun's rays are falling visibly upon your head and chest. Inhale that golden-white light so that it fills your lungs from the bottom up **[pause for inhale]**. Let it gather all the dirt, all the tensions, all the sickness within you, then release your breath **[pause]**. Watch as the light leaves your body, a dark brown or black color and returns to the earth. That is your cold being carried away **[pause]**.

Continue breathing in the Sun's golden light. It never runs out of warmth or comfort. Then exhale the dirty light, releasing it to the earth. Repeat this visualization until the light that enters is the same color as the light you exhale. **[Healer pauses and watches for signs that the patient is ready to return to normal awareness. It is important that this be done slowly, so the patient retains a balanced auric field.]**

You may feel tingly all over right now—which is fine. That's just the light rejuvenating your cells. Enjoy the positive energy for a moment **[pause]**. Now, I'd like you to change the image in your mind. See yourself back in the room with me, just as you are lying now. Increase your breathing just a little—that's it, in—out—in—out. Feel your feet, your legs, your arms begin to awaken. Take another deep breath, feel your hands, your shoulders, your face, and your forehead awaken **[pause]**.

Now, slowly open your eyes, blinking several times, until you accustom yourself to the light. Don't move right away, just lie still **[pause and observe]**. When you're ready to sit up, move slowly from your center of gravity around your navel, turning to your side, then propping yourself up on one arm first **[this maintains auric balance]**.

At this point, the healer may help the patient into a fully sitting position and discuss any images or sensations he or she experienced during the meditation. This is very important for visualization. If the imagery isn't meaningful for the participant, the healing is less likely to be successful.

Healers who regularly employ visualization are people who firmly teach that "attitude is everything." Without a positive outlook, it's hard enough to handle daily living, let alone overcome sickness. Thus, retraining the mind to think in terms of whole, healthy, successful images is part of the healer's task.

PAST-LIFE REGRESSION

> Our birth is but a sleep and a forgetting: The soul that rises with us, our life's Star, Hath had elsewhere its setting, And cometh from afar: Not in entire forgetfulness, And not in utter nakedness, But in trailing clouds of glory . . .
>
> William Wordsworth[7]

Contrary to the modern aphorism, sometimes what you don't know *can* hurt you. While there are different schools of thought regarding reincarnation,[8] most agree that the

---

[7]William Wordsworth, Ode. "Intimations of Immortality," v.

[8]Some people believe that we live many lives, and that each one teaches specific lessons that our soul carries with it after death. Similarly, traumatic experiences like drowning or falling off a cliff can have residual effects, like a fear of water or heights.

Another school of thought is that these memories are really ancestral, passed down through some genetic code. In this case, we are not living multiple lives, but are instead the sum of our ancestors' experiences. This causes feelings of déjà vu, and periodic "flashbacks."

Finally, some psychologists believe that past-life experiences are really personal myths, archetypal in nature, designed specifically to provide a detached image of the subconscious. It is, in effect, one way that the mind communicates with itself in imagery to reveal important, unresolved issues.

images from this reality do have a way of influencing our lives, here and now. By examining those experiential portraits, patients can often overcome sickness or life-long obstacles because they've been put into a different, approachable framework.

Most New Age healers working with regression therapy are doing so to uncover experiences from patients' former existences that are currently having an adverse affect on their lives. Past-life regression includes various techniques for rediscovering the root patterns of our spirit. To achieve this goal, hypnosis is one of the most frequently used methods. Hypnosis acts as does a tap in the keg of the eternal soul—it releases the froth of memories stored therein.

The idea is to provide the patient with a relaxed frame of mind through which the resulting images flow freely. From this vantage point, the subject reviews the past in a detached manner, with their present-day mind and awareness, as one watches a movie! In truth, the beginning stages of past-life regression are almost identical to guided meditation and visualization as shown above.

This time, however, once patients are relaxed, the therapist starts guiding them backward in time. Once they arrive at a past-life scenario, the therapist asks simple questions, none of which are leading, so the past-life experience unfolds naturally. Afterward, the portrait gets discussed in detail so that integration and understanding occurs.

For example, if someone has a fear of swimming, they may discover during regression that they drowned in a recent incarnation. This memory is still very close to the surface, so it manifests as an "unfounded" phobia. Sometimes knowing this is all it takes to disperse the problem.

In cases where it's not that simple, the therapist may choose to rescript the memory so that the patient experiences a positive ending to the story. The visionary capacity of the human creature has been vastly underestimated. When a patient receives an alternate snapshot of reality, it can then be added to the subconscious gallery of images, helping change the subsequent internal reactions to that event. Additionally, the post-session therapy enhances the patient's self knowledge.[9]

A PSYCHOLOGIST'S PERSPECTIVE by Arawn Machia[10]

In considering past-life regression for anyone, the most important question to ask is "why." If there is no real need for regression, I will not perform one. This is a spiritual procedure that should be approached with spiritual sensitivity. When it seems that regression may be helpful in gaining perspective unavailable during normal waking states, it is still undertaken with sensible caution. Not everyone is ready to suddenly find themselves in unfamiliar surroundings wearing a different face. Slow gentleness is important.

Additionally, it matters little if the patient is actually experiencing a past life, or simply going through a mental exercise that allows their subconscious to teach them something. What matters, ultimately, are the results—how they feel afterward about their problems, how positively they face life from that day forward. Some people have tremendous results from only one session; others need many months of regression to find the root of their difficulties; still others don't really want to face those roots. The first two types of people usually experience a fair level of success from regression, while the third will never be helped because they aren't ready.

Finally, after the session, integration is vitally important. Any therapist who neglects this step has basically wasted the entire session. People need to discuss their experiences and put them into

---

[9]As a point of interest, similar therapies are used by healers to uncover and resolve experiences in *this* life that adversely affected the patient.

[10]Used by permission. Arawn Machia is an accredited psychologist and spiritual councilor who speaks regularly on this subject, Reiki and Stregheria, around the country. He may be reached for more information by writing the author of this book through the publisher.

*perspective. They also need realistic expectations to take with them
into "real life."*

Whether symbolic in nature, or an actual experience being
relived as noted above, many psychologists are accepting
past-life regression as a viable tool for improving their patient's mental health. For more information call or write:

Athanasy, Inc.
Box 6336
Charlottesville, VA 22906
Phone: 804-973-2611
Fax: 804-975-2799

REBIRTHING

If one reviews various belief systems around the world, the
concept of rebirthing is not really innovative. Monks in the
Middle Ages often shaved their heads to signal the beginning of a new life. Nuns accepted shorter tresses and head
coverings for much the same purpose. In the 1960s, hippies
made long hair into a statement of revolutionary change,
and from the 1970s forward we heard fundamental Christians talking about the need to be "born again."

In all instances, something happens to signal transformation from one state to another, from one way of thinking
and believing to a wholly fresh vantage point. This is effectively the essence of rebirthing—to return to the womb and
work out any contrary feelings associated with that experience, then to be reborn with an improved outlook.

Rebirthing is often left in the hands of emotional care-
givers. Generally, rebirthing overcomes deep-seated emotional trauma versus actual physical problems. Nonetheless,
those same emotional traumas can cause very real physical

manifestations. In this case, pain relievers and physical manifestors may work with rebirthing as well.

The question that comes to the forefront of any discussion on rebirthing is why reliving one's birth should be mentally or physically beneficial at all. For that answer, I turned to the information shared with me by the midwives in Part II, chapter 15. Over the last century, up until recently, the process of birth had become terribly clinical. Pregnancy was treated like a disease, with all the flash and fanfare of technology, but very few humanizing, psychological, or spiritual dimensions. Frederick LeBoyer was one of the first to object to this approach in the mid-1970s, reminding us that the perinatal experience can be important to the development of both child and parent.[11]

From the records of hypnotherapists and interviews with young children, it is obvious that our brain stores the birth experience in its filing cabinet. Periodically, shadows of that record may haunt our daily reality. For example, someone retrieved by forceps at birth may experience a phobia about being grabbed suddenly. Returning to the source of their fear may be the exact prescription necessary for overcoming that problem.

During rebirthing, people may relive traumas from their early childhood as part of the staged process of regression. As with the past lives, it is easier for patients to see themselves and their experiences at younger ages in this relaxed, safe environment. Therapists believe this acts as a cathartic experience that also benefits the healing process.

A final note: Most people agree that meditation is but one part of successful therapy. A patient frequently needs other

---

[11]Stanislav Grof, *The Adventure of Self Discovery* (Albany, NY: State University of New York Press, 1988), p. 264.

supplements, including exercise and dietary guidance, to obtain long-lasting wellness. Nonetheless, at least 40–60 percent of all therapeutic benefits can be attributed to caring, loving treatment by hands-on healing, including meditative guidance.

15

Spiritual Midwifery

*In 1975 I became a spiritual midwife whose main tools are my faith in
the naturalness of birth, my healing hands and word medicine. My
promise as a spiritual midwife is to honor the journey, be attentive to
what presents itself, to remind a mother by my presence that she already
knows how to give birth . . . to respond to my original calling—to be
Keeper of the Gate. My responsibility as a healer is returning any
projections of power upon me to the family I am serving . . . Humility,
Patience, Trust, Integrity—these qualities are essential to the spiritual
midwifery practice. Healing one mother is healing the Earth.*

—Jeannine Parvati Baker

IN THIS ONE BRIEF PARAGRAPH, JEANNINE P. BAKER
summed up the essence of spiritual midwifery and high-
lighted its counseling aspects. In recent years, there has
been a revival of midwifery. Ms. Baker is but one of the talented authors to educate us, not only about this art, but
about the spiritual nature of pregnancy and ways of achieving gentle births.[1]

Women in every society have helped other women give
birth. These people were not trained in any way, other than
through what experience and other female relatives offered. Birth came where and when nature dictated: without
hospitals, without sterilization, and without a great deal of
commotion. It was, after all, a natural thing.

Some of the greatest minds in history have discussed
the role of the midwife in their societies. This indicates two
things to the modern researcher. First, that midwifery,

---

[1]Jeannine Parvati Baker is the author of *Hygieia: A Woman's Herbal, Conscious Conception, and Prenatal Yoga*. She is the founder of Hygieia College
for Spiritual Midwifery. She can be contacted at Hygieia College, P.O.
Box 398, Monroe, UT 84754-0398.

while somewhat rudimentary at its early stages, was a very honorable profession. Second, that, even though midwifery was a "woman's job," it was nonetheless distinguished. Aristotle, for example, said that a good midwife has a lady's hand, a hawk's eye, and a lion's heart. I think any modern midwife would agree wholeheartedly.

Mind you, those practicing midwifery were rarely aware of such noble concepts. Theirs was a folk tradition, passed down from mother to daughter through careful memorization. As such, much of the early transcripts regarding midwifery are steeped heavily in superstition. They also give us our first glimpse into how religion, spirituality, folk wisdom, and midwifery combined.

For example, Roman midwives swept the threshold of a laboring woman's home to drive malevolent spirits away before proceeding with their work. If a rabbit crossed the path of a woman who was near her due date, Irish midwives would recommend that she immediately tear her dress. This ensured the baby would not be born "hare-lipped." In Scotland, it was common for midwives to place a piece of iron beneath a laboring woman's bed to protect her and the baby from fairy mischief. Malaysian midwives lit fires to protect their patients from evil spirits.

When Christianity became more prevalent, this intermingling of symbolic ritual with treatment did not abate. It simply changed form to suit the new God and his followers. One 15th-century charm from Australia instructs that the following words be written on cloth and laid on the stomach of a laboring woman:

> From a man, a man; from a virgin, a virgin; the lion of the tribe of Judah conquers; Mary bore Christ; Elizabeth although sterile, John the Baptist. I adjure thee, infant, by Father, Son, and Holy Ghost, whether male or female, that thou issue forth from thy mother's body. Be thou empty! Be thou empty!

Another charm used by midwives in Ulster (given below), while totally Christian in its wording, includes all the earmarks of magic. This was written in fresh wax, then tied beneath the right foot of the mother. During the Anglo-Saxon period (and earlier) the right side of the body ruled "goodness." Wax acted as a seal to secure the power of the words. The midwives might mark a cross on the outside corners of the laboring woman's home while reciting the charm as an incantation:

> *There are four corners to her bed*
> *four angels at her head:*
> *Matthew, Mark, Luke and John,*
> *God bless the bed that she lies on.*
> *New moon, new mon, God bless me,*
> *God bless this house and family.*[2]

European midwives were popular until the Renaissance. Then, slowly, as modern medical techniques developed, they were integrated into this system under a physician's supervision. Unfortunately, with this supervision an odd attitude developed wherein pregnancy began to be treated like an illness.

For a while, it seemed that approaches to pregnancy and childbirth were doomed to remain impersonal and unfeeling. During the 1950s, for example, fathers were regularly left out of the entire birth process. Until recently, children rarely discussed their new sibling until after the baby was home, and never participated in birth, unless it was an unexpected home delivery.

---

[2]Both these charms appear in *WitchCraft and Magic* by Venetia Newall (London: Hamlyn, 1974), pp. 122–123. The second charm is also referred to in *Folk Medicine* by William George Black (New York: Burt Franklin, 1883), p. 128. The form of the charm is exactly the same in both texts.

It is uncertain what exactly led to this emotionally sterile approach to pregnancy. Perhaps in our zealousness to ensure "safe" births and the longevity of our species, we accidentally forsook the essence of what birth represents. It is the ultimate human creative expression, as old as the species, and as organic as a daisy. So, the question remains, why all the fuss?

Yes, it is important to take sensible precautions with prenatal care and the birth itself. However, this is not just another clinical procedure. Metaphysically, the family and midwife are welcoming a soul to the Earth plane. With this in mind, harsh lights, plastic gloves, and machinery seem awkward and out of place. The midwife offers families a chance to reclaim the naturalness of birth without necessarily shedding all the safety nets of modern medicine. To illustrate, here are my own birth stories:

Karl and Samantha

Just nine years ago, my son Karl was born. At that time, I was given very few options. The hospital required *an IV, an external and internal monitor, pubic shaving, and a number of other procedures that I really didn't want. By the time they were done, I felt a bit like Frankenstein's monster, hooked up to numerous tubes and wires. There was no way to be comfortable, and I was not allowed a birthing room because the baby was a little early.*

To make matters worse, the baby had problems breathing. I never even got to hold Karl until he was five days old. During that time, I had to pump my breast milk and bring it to the hospital. By the time he was healthy enough to come home, Karl was a stranger to me. I didn't know what to do or how to feel—and there was no one to give me advice. I was miserable for about a month!

Thankfully, by the time my daughter Samantha was born last year, much had changed. My health provider offered a midwife, whose strength and encouragement during labor were nothing short of amazing. This time, every part of my birth experience was planned by myself and my husband. The midwife made suggestions when we had questions, but always complied with our decisions. The whole experience was more positive, so that by the time we took Samantha home, I was really ready to be her mother.

One week later, I received three separate calls. One from the midwife, one from my nurse, and one from a lactation specialist, just to be sure both the baby and I were "okay." These people were taking part in our well-being as a family—a gesture for which I will always be thankful.

What this change indicates to me is that finally, over the last decade, women's voices have been heard. We have spoken out about our bodies and reproductive choices. The number of legally practicing midwives has grown proportional to the swelling desire among families to make birth a unified, supportive experience. Colleges for midwifery have developed across the country, and the number of home births by choice are increasing.[3]

While some doctors find this new attention to "naturalness" somewhat disturbing, the Mothering Prenatal Healthcare Index showed that infants have lower mortality rates in countries where midwives are the principal birth attendants.[4] Women report they feel more at ease with a midwife, because the midwife doesn't treat pregnancy so clinically. Most women will have shorter labors, use less pain medication (if any), have fewer forceps deliveries, and experience fewer Caesarean sections under a midwife's or professional birth assistant's care.[5]

---

[3]According to a study conducted by the Center for Birth and Human Development (Berkeley, CA), there is no statistical benefit to choosing a hospital versus homebirth. These findings seem substantiated by other studies, and actually the results improve when the mother is attended by an experienced midwife.

[4]*Mothering*, Fall 1993, p. 45.

[5]"The Professional Birth Assistant," *Special Delivery*, Vol. 16, Winter 1992–1993, p. 2.

Today, the International Federation of Gynecology and Obstetrics defines a midwife as a person who has studied a recognized midwifery program and met the qualifications for graduation. A midwife gives supervision before, during, and after the pregnancy, provides advice and guidance, may take part in emergency medical measures, and works with the family on education regarding childcare and birth control. Noncertified midwives may or may not be legal, depending on the area in which they practice. This may leave the spiritual midwife in a quandary if he or she lacks accreditation.

Some healthcare providers have nurse-midwives available to pregnant women who evidence no signs of physical difficulties. While these women do not necessarily have spiritual goals in mind, they are definitely sensitive to physical ones. Additionally, there are people in the New Age community who are training to be licensed midwives so they can provide families with spiritual encouragement along with professional advice.

I turned to just such a person during my second pregnancy. Being hesitant to face labor again after the first experience, I called her, hoping for any good advice. Kym was patient, understanding, helpful, and encouraging. She explained how having a midwife would change my birth experience in detail, and she was 100 percent correct. Kym sent the following reflections on her work.[6]

The Midwife Serves Women

While some midwives are merely obstetricians without medical sanction, most are different in that they consider it essential to protect

[6]Kym is a Certified Childbirth Educator for informed birth through ALACE (Association of Labor Assistants and Childbirth Educators). She has collected a tremendous amount of material on natural childbirth, homebirth, and spiritual midwifery. For more information, you may write her at Box 178, Pentwater, MI 49449. Please send SASE.

the sacredness of birth. They honor and respect both the mother and the new soul. There are as many different kinds of spiritual midwives as there are paths.

The word midwife means "with women." The duties of a midwife are varied, and perhaps even more so for those spiritually guided. We are observers[7] who listen intuitively, check blood pressure, take temperatures, watch the baby's progress and generally maintain a watchful eye on all birth participants (not just the mother). If tensions increase, the source needs to be found and quieted. A very observant spiritual midwife can often detect difficulties long before mechanical devices, because she is already attuned to all aspects of that birth.

In addition, the midwife may take on the roles of childbirth educator, friend, counselor, maid, laundry person, masseuse, chef, lactation consultant, and dietary advisor. In short, whatever *the birthing couple needs to have a pure birth. Midwives do not "manage" a birth, they serve women.[8] They do not deliver a baby—only mothers can do that. Instead, they help receive the child.*

Most of all, the spiritual midwife recognizes that pregnancy is not an illness. Birth should be an empowering event. The mother has carried the entire power of creation within her for nine months. She is now becoming a channel for universal energy, and needs to be aware of that wonder—of her own self-worth. This awareness helps give the mother confidence in her own ability to give birth, and to care for that soul when it arrives.

---

[7]A German midwifery text of 1513, cited in Janet Isaccs Ashford's pamphlet, *Midwives* (1988), says: "The Midwife herself shall sit before the labouring woman and shall diligently observe and wait . . . also the midwife must instruct and comfort the party, not only refreshing her with good meate and drinke, but also with sweet words."

[8]While the role of midwife has traditionally been left in the hands of women, more men are now entering the nurse-midwife profession, with mixed reception by the public. Some feel that it's good for more men to have an understanding of gentle births, while others feel men cannot fully comprehend the woman's role. Both schools of thought have merit.

In terms of drawbacks, the major one is being at odds with the medical establishment. Midwifery is more accepted now than ever, but many midwives still have to swim "up stream" to gain that acceptance. This sometimes causes burnout. Additionally, it makes educating your patients twice as difficult—you must replace their fears with confidence and show them that midwifery is a natural, time-honored tradition.

So, the job of the spiritual midwife is akin to what midwives have been doing since the dawn of time: giving aid and support to their patients. The only major difference here is the addition of another dimension, one sensitive to the metaphysical world and ideals. This does not lessen the importance of any other portion of the midwife equation; it simply balances them into a wholeness that welcomes the spirit being born.

Welcoming is a process that begins before labor for the family, and then is intensified by the birth. To help the mother, some midwives provide focus by chanting, special breathing techniques, visualizations, or symbols. Each is designed with that mother in mind to help her birth experience be positive and empowering.

Of these, chanting can be doubly effective since it already uses breath, has elements of word magic, and can facilitate trance-like states. Chanting naturally increases with the labor pains, acting as an emotional release. It can also become a cry to the universe for an open pathway (spiritually and physically).

For example, one midwife might suggest using the sound "Ah" (as in Anma, or mother) as an aid. This is a natural sound which escapes the lips when pain occurs, but it also carries the vibration of motherhood. During times of rest, another sound or phrase can be used for relaxation, a sound such as "AUM"—the affirmation of existence. With the midwife beside her firmly guiding her, the mother can use these or other tools to maintain her focus, and let divine energy flow into delivery.

Immediately after the birth, the midwife checks the baby's health, then gives the child into its mother's arms for feeding. Other family members are encouraged to stroke the child and whisper reassuring words. This improves emotional bonding and makes everyone active participants in this ritual of life called birth. By this time, the relationship between midwife and mother is very strong. They may laugh or cry together, and for a moment the spiritual midwife is an integral part of that special family unit.

I think that spiritual midwives have one of the most wonderful (and sometimes difficult) jobs. They are the gate keepers for future generations. Midwives are teaching families across the world how to open their hearts and souls to a sacred experience. They are helping women reclaim the holiness of their bodies and bodily choices. And, in some cases, they help those who lose children to grieve, let go, and heal. Slowly, spiritual midwives will take their rightful place beside women again, welcomed by a needy medical and magical community. For many families, this change can not happen soon enough.

RESOURCE MATERIALS FOR MIDWIFERY

Most of these books are available through large bookstores. Another source for them is Cascade Birthing, 141 Commercial St. NE, Salem, OR 97301; 1-800-443-9942. While there are many others available, I believe this list will get you started with healthy "food for thought" if you're considering, or practicing, this art.

Artemis Speaks: BAC Stories & Natural Childbirth Information by Nan Koehler (Caesarean Sections).
Birth without Violence, Frederick Leboyer.

Breastfeeding, Mary Renfrew, Fisher, and Arms.

Healing Yourself During Pregnancy, Joy Gardner (Nutrition).

Heart & Hands: A Midwife's Guide to Pregnancy and Birth, Elizabeth Davis.

Homebirth, Sheila Kitzinger.

Special Delivery, Rahima Baldwin (Birthing Methods).

Spiritual Midwifery, Ina May Gaskin.

Wise Woman's Herbal for the Childbearing Year, Susun Weed.

Witches, Midwives & Nurses: A History of Women Healers, Barbara Ehrenreich and Deirdre English.

16

Reiki

All we need do is want to achieve something
great, and then simply do it. Never think of
failure, for what we think will come about.
—Maharishi Mahesh Yogi

REIKI[1] ORIGINATED IN JAPAN AS A SYSTEM OF LAYING
on of hands to improve a patient's physical flow of energy.
Reiki employs specific hands-on systems to renew physical
and spiritual well-being. More than this, however, Reiki is a
way of thinking and being as a supplement to the body's
natural way of healing. Reiki practitioners encourage their
patients to open themselves to understanding the nature of
Spirit and its energy, so that inner harmony is supple-
mented along with health.

Reiki practitioners recognize that they must live and
act in harmony with all created things. It is simple and
holistic: one may feel love, experience rapture, and renew
health by maintaining that harmony. To these healers, it is
no accident that the word "bliss" and "bless" are similar—
they are, in fact, part of one another.

---

[1]Reiki translates roughly to "universal life power," or "universal spirit."

HISTORY

While probably having far older roots, Reiki had its beginnings in the mid-19th century with Dr. Mikao Usui. Dr. Usui
began studying rehabilitative systems that use sounds and
emblems as a key component in the late 1800s. Over the
next twenty-seven years, this study continued. Finally, after
entering a Zen monastery and a spiritual retreat, Usui
began using sacred sounds and symbols for healing. To try
his ideas, he spent seven years treating the street people of
Kyoto, then began traveling to teach others the technique
that we now know as Reiki.

Dr. Usui outlined the basic ethical guidelines for Reiki
masters:

Bear no worry into treatment, or into life;
Carry no anger;
Always remember to honor your elders and teachers;
Earn an honest living;
Live gratefully.

In truth, I believe he devised a very sound approach to living for anyone, not just Reiki practitioners!

By 1982, the Reiki Alliance formed (a statement of
purpose for this group can be found on-line at http://cy-
bertap.com/date/alliance.html). This alliance advocates
Dr. Usui's guidelines and tiered teaching to encourage
hands-on experiential healers. For example, to an un-
trained homeowner, piping may seem to be functioning
perfectly well, whereas to a trained plumber, all manner of
warning signs might exist. The teaching period for the
Reiki Mastery turns the homeowner into the experienced
plumber through time and practice (see also section on
credentials, to follow).

Since the early 1980s, Reiki practitioners and associations have grown in number. There are now registered
Reiki Masters in areas as diverse as Hawaii, Canada, Malta,

and Ireland, just to name a few. Seminars are held around the world, offering various degrees to students. Regional conferences are also starting to be assembled so that Reiki healers, and those who would be so, as well as other healers with harmonic viewpoints, can exchange ideas and information. For a contact address, see the end of this chapter.

THE PROCESS

Beyond ethics, Usui taught that Reiki responds to what each patient needs most. The session often begins with some water or tea for the patient to aid the cleansing process (and also to improve relaxation). Practitioners remove any jewelry, cleanse their hands, make sure the patient is comfortable, and ensure that the next half hour will pass undisturbed.

Next, healers begin laying their hands on a patient (or in close proximity thereto) with the fingers closed. They then open themselves to universal energy, staying in designated regions for three to five minutes each. The seven designated areas are:

Shoulders;
Top of the head;
Forehead and base of the head;
Seventh vertebrae and throat;
Evenly on the breastbone and back;
Evenly on the stomach and back;
Evenly on the lower stomach and lower back.

These are not hard-and-fast guidelines, however. Reiki does allow for inspired flexibility.

During Reiki, the patient may experience sensations of cold or warmth, see visions, have unexpected emotions surface, or even manifest physical responses like trembling. No matter the patient's experience, however, the goal of the Reiki master is therapeutic—to return the body-mind-spirit to an orderly state. Therefore, Reiki is a tradition that will work very well with just about any other methodology, as long as the goal is similar.

For someone who cannot be present, Reiki can still be effective, based on the idea that every thought can, and does, touch those to whom we send it. Think of energy as a universal telephone through which you can dial the right number in your thoughts. Having a photograph or personal items from the individual helps, but just their name will do. In this case, it is best for recipients to lie down at a designated time and meditate so they're more open and receptive to the healing. This should not be done without permission.

Reiki also works well on children, animals, or plants, the only difference being that the amount of time for a complete session is much shorter, totaling around ten minutes. If an animal is skittery, try allowing them to sleep in your lap during a session. Fish can be held in their aquarium, allowing the water to act as an "auric" field. Other, larger animals respond positively to touches behind the ears and neck. In this way, a Reiki healer can literally touch any living thing, from people to the whole planet. What could be more "whole-istic?"

Once you learn the techniques of Reiki, also consider allowing that energy to flow into your daily meals, then internalize your bliss!

REIKI by Arawn Machia[2]

One of the greatest advantages of practicing Reiki is becoming a conduit for Universal Energy. This way, there is no direct drain on

[2]See also Part II, chapter 3, "Auric Cleansing and Balancing."

the practitioner. In order for healers to be truly effective, however, they must take time to attune themselves to that energy. This time acts like insulation for the practitioner, so the ensuing power flows without diversions to where it is most needed.

A second advantage is that Reiki is nonintrusive. It is not necessary to interrupt personal space when interacting with the aura. Obviously, if a patient is more open, it assists the process, but ultimately a person's aura can be affected from across a room if necessary.

Third, it is virtually impossible to overdo a Reiki healing. During treatments, there is an interplay between three energies: the patient's, healer's, and that of the Universe. Often the healer will feel drawn to the Universal Powers just before a session begins, then sense that flow withdraw as it ends. Even if they don't, any excess energy just grounds itself out.

The time taken for treatments varies according to the needs of the individual. On average, it takes an hour for a full-body treatment, during which more time may be spent in specific areas of need. Nonetheless, imbalance is often a global matter, so doing full-body work generally produces better results than a quicker, localized session.

Afterward, most patients report feeling more peaceful and connected. This is because Reiki realigns the subtle bodies on various levels of the aura, thereby improving the body's natural healing capacity. Additionally, some people experience visions, feel vibrations or other sensations, or have sudden emotional releases. Consequently Reiki is very effective for helping the spiritual/emotional dis-ease that often manifests in physical conditions.

Yet, I must caution both potential healers and those seeking treatment that they really must have confidence and a personal connection to a technique to achieve lasting success. With confidence in hand, Reiki may be used alone or in concert for truly remarkable results. Better still, healers will find themselves experiencing positive psychic, physical, and emotional changes. These changes reflect the spiritual revolution that's inspired by the

Universal Life Force—the power that has now basically become a partner with the healer in the quest for wholeness.

CREDENTIALS FOR REIKI

While the basic ideas of Reiki are accessible to anyone, the Reiki technique is not something that you can learn on your own, at least not if you wish to pursue mastery. It must be studied with a recognized master, and includes three degrees for total proficiency. In the United States, it is commonly called the Radiance Technique, and it must be studied with a master, going through seven degrees to become proficient.

This tiered teaching system is very specific, beginning with a basic understanding of energy, proceeding to the laying on of hands, and culminating in techniques for transferring energy to oneself and others. One side benefit of this process is that, the more healers use Reiki, the more universal energy flows through them. So, they inevitably experience personal growth, too.

Higher levels of study must be approved by a master. In these classes, healers learn to do absentee work, as well as how to improve their own style within the Reiki guidelines. At this juncture, healers may start to teach others in order to fund the expense of becoming a master, which is quite costly. This is understandable when one considers the years and sacrifice necessary to attain this level of knowledge.

REIKI RESULTS

The goal of Reiki is to empower the patient by channeling universal energy; Reiki does not use massage. Instead, the healer's hands remain passive, allowing the universal power to be the active, empowering force, along with the patient's own healing capacity. Most treatments seem effective in treating tension, improving creativity, and promoting self-love.

In most cases, once this is achieved, the patient suddenly finds they have the drive and vision necessary to overcome repression and follow their dreams. Reiki helps re-establish balance in all bodily energies, cleanses impurities, and generally relaxes patients who have trouble relaxing.

For further information write:
Center for Reiki Training
29209 Northwestern Hwy. #592
Southfield, MI 48034
Phone: 1-800-332-8112
Fax: 248-948-9534
E-Mail: center@reiki.org

Reiki Healing Institute
449 Santa Fe Dr., Box 303
Encinitas, CA 92024
Phone: 619-436-1865
Fax: 619-436-6875
E-Mail: empower@webtv.net

17

Sound Therapy

There is in souls a sympathy with sounds;
And, as the mind is pitched the ear is pleased
With melting airs, or martial, brisk, or grave:
Some chord in unison with what we hear,
Is touched within us, and the heart replies.
—William Cowper

RELIGIONS AROUND THE WORLD USE SOUND AS AN integral part of worship. Westerners pray or sing aloud; Easterners may meditate and recite the AUM chant. In the background, traditional music can be heard in both cultures.

Many writers and philosophers at various stages in history have discussed the music of the spheres, universal energy, the resonance of creation, the power of words, and marching to a different drummer. Legend even goes so far as to claim that Greek musicians could know a person, or effect a cure, through one note. Why? A good portion of the importance placed on sound, no matter the era or culture, comes from human usage and reactions.

Even among animals, tonal qualities convey worlds of meaning. Sounds indicate the full measure and scope of human emotion, and have direct repercussions on the self, the listener, and the overall environment. Consider for a moment how the atmosphere of a room changes when two people begin to argue and you have a good example of how sound transforms energy as it vibrates outward from the source. Similarly, people who restrain natural noises like sneezing, crying, or roaring in pain, will sometimes experience dis-ease from the sound being internalized.

DIAGNOSIS

The first thing to which a sound therapist listens is a patient's voice. This is a strong indicator of emotion, stability, and personality. Shy people often exhibit thin voices, while those who are under stress speak harshly or with a cracked tonal quality. An enthusiastic, healthy individual will have a strong, steady, and uplifting voice. So, in effect, our words indicate not only what type of energy we are sending out, but what we have accepted into ourselves!

GOOD VIBRATIONS

Sound is a powerful tool for changing individual and collective consciousness—just watch a rock concert sometime to verify this fact. It has the potential to break down social, religious, and philosophical barriers by being a universal language to which all living things respond. Yet knowing exactly which sounds are "good sounds" for an individual patient is not an easy task.

Sound is vibrational in nature, which is exactly what makes it a perfect medium for holistic healing, although one that must be used carefully. When trained opera singers create a tone at a high enough pitch that resonates exactly with a glass, the glass shatters. Healers don't want their vibrational work to result in a physical, spiritual, or emotional "shattering."

This is where sensitivity to each patient and what sounds are most beneficial for their condition becomes essential. Each vibration symbolizes something specific to the subconscious and spirit of an individual. Some music makes us happy, some tones make us sad, and others pass by us unnoticed. Additionally, healers must be certain of their personal motivations and moods so that no negative "vibes" get accidentally translated into the procedure.

Thankfully, there do seem to be a few generalizations that can be made (with caution). For example, New Age music seems to soothe the sixth and seventh chakras, while jazz stimulates these same regions. Root chakras are energized by upbeat music, almost literally igniting dance and movement. Drumming can affect any chakra just by changing the rhythm and presentation. Soft music aids digestion and bursts of sound improve lethargy.

Whatever the final sounds chosen, however, sound therapists follow a simple progression for their work. They begin with a prelude of sound that prepares the individual, followed by a body of music that transports the listener to the appropriate level of awareness so healing may begin. And the finale brings the real world back into focus and provides closure.

THE PATIENT'S PART

Our society frowns on what it regards as inappropriate sound. By inappropriate, what we really mean is a sound that makes *us* uncomfortable when we hear it—no matter how much good it may do the person from whom it was uttered. Someone who regularly suppresses sound may eventually become ill, according to the basic formula expression = emotion = energy. Restrained energy has to be housed somewhere in the auric field, so someone who keeps silent rather than speaking the truth, for example, may experience a sore throat.

One part of sound therapy is showing patients that sound is a natural part of life and teaching them how to release society-trained self-consciousness so that they can also release their sickness. Sound therapists discourage patients from verbally or mentally associating themselves with a named sickness, because naming things gives them power. Even the ancients were aware of this, often giving the inflicted person a new name temporarily to fool any malevolent spirit hovering nearby.

Sound therapists encourage patients to find their own set of healing sounds that they can use and carry with them anywhere. If possible, this personal set of tones follows melodic or rhythmic patterns to help commit it to memory. Beyond this, the value of silence is not overlooked in this art. Quiet time to meditate, pray, and inspect personal feelings is also strongly encouraged. Patients, however, must take responsibility for regularly integrating these tools into their lives to maintain wellness.

THE HEALING SONG

The sound of the soul is totally unique within each person. Those with trained spiritual senses can recognize this music and use it to know a person's overall bearing. Sound therapists use this attunement to recognize sickness and then determine the best tones to reverse the problem.

This results in what is called a healing song—an individually devised set of sounds that envelop the patient in harmonious tones. These sounds may equate to a song, chant, mantra, tones, drumming, or notes played upon a musical instrument. The idea is to help patients readjust their personal vibrations to those of the universe—rather like a tuning fork.

In most cases, a "healing song" (which may or may not have actual "musical" qualities) has a similar beginning and end for each patient, but the middle modulates depending on patients' needs. This transformation is not something healers plan, but one which they allow to be guided by higher powers.

If a person is deaf, this does not mean the healing song cannot affect them. Deaf people are very sensitive to vibrations, out of necessity. Also, healing songs don't have to be used just on people—animals, plants, and the planet itself all benefit from such soothing sounds. Earth healers may find this a tremendously useful technique to learn to better attune themselves with specific ecospheres (see Part II, chapter 8, "Earthly Realms").

FINDING YOUR HEALING SONG

Your healing song has probably been with you for a very long time. Perhaps you hummed a little tune when you were sad or hurt as a child. Maybe you hum a ditty when you're alone and it makes you feel better. If you have a refrain like this, try singing it to someone else when they're out of sorts and see what happens. Chances are, it will help them, too. If so, this is your healing song. If not, try this exercise.

If it is physically possible, fast for a day, then go to a quiet place where you will not be disturbed. Allow your heart and mind to settle until peacefulness surrounds you within and without. Next, slowly begin enunciating each vowel aloud. Fill your diaphragm with air first, letting the air carry the sound. Feel how each vowel activates a different chakra; *e* is the first, *o* is the second, *i* is the third, *u* is the fourth and *ah* is the fifth. This last sound is particularly potent for releasing pain.

When you've done this once or twice, sit quietly and see what sounds come to mind. If you wait for a long time and nothing occurs, try drumming a little, using slow, varied rhythms for about seven minutes. Then be quiet again. When sounds come, they will seem familiar, but not necessarily from any music or language to which you're accustomed.

Mystics have always claimed that forms of language other than those we use exist, so consider this a spiritual translation of linguistics into a potent symbolic form of self-expression. Don't try to find more sounds than you get initially; just make sure you remember those received. This music will grow of its own accord, depending on the need and your openness.

If this exercise proves fruitless for you, don't despair. Healing songs can come to you any time, anywhere, and may even appear in your dreams. If this happens and you wake up, hum your song a couple of times before returning to bed so you remember it.

Finally, healing songs do not have to be uttered aloud to work. There are circumstances in life that require silent communication. Thinking one's healing song is just as powerful as voicing it outwardly, except that you may find you have to project more to release that energy.

OTHER SONGS

There is an old saying that "music soothes the savage beast." In sound therapy, healers apply sound to soothe physical ailments by adjusting auric energies first, then slowly moving the soundwave inward until it touches the molecular level. All life resonates, and a sound therapist is closely attuned to that vibration within themselves and others, which is why music makes a perfect vehicle for this technique.

Life-song: A life-song is similar to a healing song in that it has been with you since birth. Unlike the healing song, however, this is not music to share; it is your power song. When sung or chanted, this song increases the energy in the auric field and dispels negativity. Thus, the life-song is a valuable tool for accepting, empowering, and maintaining healing arts. In fact, *all healers* can use this music to prepare themselves for their work.

Those who understand how life-songs work can become guides for patients who need to find this music in order to rediscover their own sense of sacredness and connection to Spirit. Many people today feel lost in the crowd and overwhelmed by responsibilities. Knowing and singing your life-song is a way to reaffirm self-worth, individuality, and personal vision. Regularly reciting your life-song also improves health and emotional well-being.

To find your life-song, try going into a quiet, dark room and watching the flame of a candle. Fire is intimately symbolic of creation and life's essence. Breathe slowly, and listen. Your life-song may not have any words, and it may take several attempts over time to discover it. Frequently, the life-song manifests during periods of drastic transformation to help you integrate change. Once found, life-songs should be sung as loudly as possible as a confirmation of life itself. They are also a very useful aid for vision quests.

On a personal note, some people believe the life-song never changes—that it is like a harmonic chord that echoes the immortal soul. I agree, in part, that a certain refrain from your life-song will always stay with you. But, since the soul is hopefully always growing and changing, you may find that, one day, your life-song also transforms to reflect this maturation. If it does, don't let this worry you. It is just an outward manifestation of inward evolution.

Saga Songs: Another technique sound therapists may teach patients is how to make up songs that help them to begin positively using experiences from the recent past to empower the future. With life moving so quickly today, when changes occur, most people feel pressured to just "get on with it." Then we idly wonder why certain cycles constantly reappear in our lives.

In our hurry to cope, we never really accept life's lessons and employ them in our spiritual growth. Saga songs help us bridge this gap through words and lyrics, sound and silence. Here, sound therapists remind us to stop for a moment and find the words or tones to express inner evolution. In the process, our own awareness of this transformation helps ignite energy for anything we hope to accomplish.

In the end, sound therapists are really working with our auric energies. By adding specific vibrations to those of a patient, the healer begins massaging the auric envelope into a balanced, harmonious whole. This envelope then encourages the body and mind to function at an improved capacity, thereby aiding the natural ability to heal.

The results this engenders in the patient vary with each case. Some patients experience an involuntary physical response, like itching or sneezing. This is actually very positive, as it indicates the release of some unresolved issues. Other people may feel odd bursts of energy or emotions, see flashes from their past, or smell an odd fragrance in the air. This phenomenon is called synesthesia, and it happens because sound also activates our memory centers.

For more information on sound healing call or write:

Casa de Maria
Musical Massage
1195 Monticello Rd.
Napa, CA 94558
Phone: 888-262-8348

APPENDIX A
HEALER, HEAL THYSELF

It is important for everyone to care for their physical well-being. For healers, this is even more true for many reasons, not the least of which is the ability to enjoy life fully. Nonetheless, when a healer is out of sorts, no matter how skilled he or she may be, the wrong kind of energy can inadvertently get projected into their patients.

For example, a wonderful woman I know told me of a trip to a chiropractor, where she suddenly felt frightened during the treatment. There was no apparent reason for her fear, yet the emotion manifested so strongly that it probably undid any good that visit may have accomplished. In this illustration, the healer allowed personal fears, misgivings, or other negativities to "spill" over into the patient's auric envelope. The patient interpreted this energy as fear, and that's all she could focus on throughout the treatment.

This story is a very good illustration of the kinds of problems inherent in metaphysically empowered healing techniques. No matter the approach, each healer is somehow channeling universal energy through the vessel of self. Just as one prefers clean pots and pans in which to prepare dinner, this energy "tastes" much better for patients when it flows through a healthy, emotionally "clean" vessel.

So, what can healers do to help themselves? Well, besides getting some decent rest, a lot depends on the problem at hand. Here is a brief overview of common maladies and fairly easy aids to get you started:

Backache

Herbal: Try a tincture of agrimony steeped in vinegar applied to the back with a long-handled loofah.

Reflexology: Since most people can reach their hands and feet, reflexology is the perfect hands-on approach for self-healing, too. Check an accurate chart for proper pressure and massage points.

Warm moisture: This is achieved by spritzing a towel thoroughly with water and warming it in a microwave or oven until steamy. Place this on the afflicted area (take care with the temperature, perhaps putting a thin cloth between your skin and the towel). If heat doesn't relieve the pain, try ice instead.

Visualization: Sit with your back against a tree and visualize that strength merging with your back and the pain pouring into the earth.

Colds and Flu

Aromatherapy: Try a mixture of mint, ginger, anise, cedar, cinnamon, and eucalyptus in a steaming potpourri. Keep the steaming aromatics in the room where you spend the most time.

Crystal therapy: Carry agate regularly to improve overall immunity.

Herbal: A tea made from one teaspoon each of eucalyptus, chamomile, orange rind, rosehips, rosemary, sage, and mint steeped in two cups of boiling water. Add honey as desired for sweetness.

Headache

Bach's flower remedy: For headaches stemming from foreboding, try oak. For stress-related headaches, use olive, and for those originating from fears or anxiety, apply aspen.

Folk remedial: Place fresh cucumber peels on your temples and lie down in a dark, quiet area.

Herbal: Raspberry-catnip tea consumed near quiet background noise, like a CD track of a gentle spring rain.

Massage: Gently rub your temples where the head and neck connect and at the base of the neck with three fingers, moving in slowly extending circles.

Lethargy

Auric balancing or cleansing: Survey your whole body spiritually to see if you can detect imbalance. If you do, visualize any excesses or deficiencies being evened out. Then burn some energetic herbs, like ginger, and use a feather to fan them into your energy field.

Common sense: This may indicate your body's struggle to ward off illness. If you've been exposed to colds or flu, try increasing your vitamin C intake and get a little extra rest. Dressing sensibly for the season, being more cautious than usual about covering your head, the area of highest heat loss. If the situation doesn't improve, try the alternatives listed below.

Diet and exercise: Increase high-energy foods like fresh fruit juices; decrease red meat; begin slowly increasing physical activity levels.

Sound therapy: Incorporate tapes, records, or CDs that contain bursts of sound into your environment. One piece of music that seems suitable to this goal is the "1812 Overture," complete with cannon fire, to propel refreshed energy. I also personally find the sounds of a Spanish guitar played by a passionate artist to be most uplifting.

Visualization: Two images seem to work fairly well. The first is envisioning white, sparkling light pouring into you, specifically near the heart chakra, then spreading throughout the body. Another good image is that of going to a well full of light-water and drinking until you can absorb no more.

Self-Image and Insecurity

Affirmations: Affirmations are positive words that engender good images and healthful vibrations in and around you. Consider the areas that seem to need the most development and focus on them one at a time. Don't overwhelm yourself with too many expectations; growth for you is no less difficult than it is for those you heal.

Aromatherapy: In this case, herbalism and aromatherapy work quite nicely together. Mix one teaspoon each of orange bergamot tea and lavender flowers in one cup of water. The smell from each inspires improved confidence, and the tea itself eases the associated tensions that come with timidity.

Silence is golden: Sometimes, when words or sounds don't seem appropriate, silence is the greatest healer. Tranquility attunes or resensitizes your life-force to that of the universe. This gives you time to collect your thoughts, calm the mental chatter, breathe and worship, and generally see things more clearly. It also allows you to reconnect with the sacred through simple things like a sighing wind, until your images of self are totally unified with that sacred energy, bringing peace within and without.

Stress and Tension Relief

Crystals: Someone once told me to go to a field, find a common, everyday-looking stone, and tell my troubles to it.

Somehow, the ancientness of that rock, and leaving it in the field when I went on my way, combined into a very effective exercise. You need not go to a field, however, if one isn't available. Just find any stone, in any convenient location from which you can turn your back, neatly leaving your problems behind you.

Mantras: Mantras are sacred prayers that may be totally personal—a reaffirmation of the self. Mystical teachers tell us these banish negativity and provide courage to the spiritual warrior to face anything, including heavy burdens. Fortitude is necessary in many other areas of our lives, too, like facing our daily routines. That inner resolution and confidence reduce stress.

Stunning simplicity: Sometimes, laughter is indeed a terrific healer. When we laugh fully and freely, it disburses negative energy quite rapidly. Try watching a humorous movie or going to a comedy club, and remember how to laugh at yourself and life once again. Just because you are a healer, doesn't mean that enlightenment comes easily. But humor always makes any rocky road a little easier to travel.

If all else fails, including conventional medicine, don't neglect to ask for help from another trained healer, in whose approach you believe and trust. Many healers I know have the most difficulty reaching out when it comes to their own needs. What they don't realize is that, by so doing, they deny the temple of their soul and thereby taint their own ability to work effectively.

Care diligently for yourself. You are your most important patient.

APPENDIX B
FINDING THE "RIGHT" HEALER

Throughout this book, I have discussed each healing technique with as much insight, balance, and caution as possible without undermining the power of faith. Yet this is only a sketch of some very intricate fields. Thus, if you cannot heal yourself, or need help with a particularly vexing problem, I urge you to investigate any individual to whom you go for aid.

How? In the interest of creating some type of guidelines, I present the following for your consideration. It may be that some healers make you feel so immediately at ease that the techniques given here are unnecessary. This appendix is not written as the proverbial hysteria generator. A great majority of people in alternative medicine are honest, caring folk.

Instead, I hope to be the voice of caution. No matter how deep and abiding your faith may be in a method, don't ignore wariness or overlook warning signs. I cannot stress enough the importance of trusting your healer's credentials, claims, and conventions. Nothing less than your personal well-being is at stake.

Office staff attitude: When you make your initial inquiry at the healer's home or office, how are you treated? Terse people who hedge your questions may have something to hide. On the other hand, professionals sometimes have bad days just like everyone else. So if you felt a little put-off by the initial phone call, try one more time to alleviate or confirm that discomfort.

If it doesn't infringe on another patient's privacy, will this healer allow you to observe some treatments, or perhaps receive a free or discounted sample treatment before subscribing to an entire series? In massage, for example, vastly different methods exist, not all of which are right for everyone. Without more information, how can you make an educated decision? Offices that are a little more open and flexible about allowing you to "test drive" their services and tour the facilities are generally those that are also more trustworthy. Note, however, that advance arrangements will probably have to be made in the interest of being sensitive to other clients' needs.

Credentials and professional associations: In metaphysical realms, these are not always a necessity. One of the most talented healers that I know of personally has no credentials to show, other than those given by the universe. Even so, this individual has made an effort to contact other healers in related fields for input and ideas. That effort is something that could be traced, if something seemed amiss.

Someone who claims to have a license or affiliations must be registered *somewhere* (note the addresses given throughout this book). If you feel ill at ease about the credentials with which you're presented, ask questions and check all references, including making phone calls to listed schools. It may take a little time to get your answers, but the peace of mind is well worth it.

Recommendations and references: If possible, get the recommendations of friends or other people that you trust, and call the healer's references. If you can't find any, look at the bulletin boards at food cooperatives and New Age stores/centers. Also check the internet! Once you find a few people who know about the healer you're seriously considering, ask them lots of questions, including those that pertain directly to your condition if that person was treated for similar problems.

Better Business Bureau: With New Age ideology coming into its own, more alternative medical businesses are being registered with the Better Business Bureau. Similarly, less reputable firms which have received complaints are listed by this organization. So, while you might not find out much, a quick call here may prove productive.

Your responsibility: If you choose to try a healer, and during the treatment something seems wrong, say so! Make yourself the principle partner in your body's wellness. Watch the response you receive from the healer. Does he or she stop and listen carefully to your concerns, then take time to explain or adjust the approach used? Or, does the healer seem insulted and put off? The first is someone for whom holistic treatment has real meaning. The second is likely only working for a paycheck.

Second opinions count: I believe this is true of any medical profession. No reputable healer squirms or fusses when you say you'd like a second opinion. Nonetheless, I really suggest *you* find someone to turn to for that opinion, instead of asking the healer's staff for suggestions. It's human nature to want to be right and, out of a sense of loyalty, the staff may steer you toward people whom they know will concur with the given findings. By having a "blind" second opinion, the feedback you receive is more likely to be balanced.

Balancing what's known with what's believed: It is quite true that the New Age is "coming of age." Even so, many alternative medical practices are still regarded as being in their infancy, no matter how ancient the origins. Consequently, it is very important that you recognize that some therapies are based more on faith than actual, verifiable proof.

To illustrate, massage therapy has been tested through carefully monitored studies and documentation and has 3,000 years of history to back it up. On the other hand, crystal therapists and auric healers still receive scowls and headshakes from those who don't trust in the techniques' validity. For a devout patient, the lack of testing matters little. Yet, reputable practitioners of such arts explain this difference to their patients *before* proceeding or accepting any type of payment.

Does the healer have sliding scale fees or payment plans: This is not a hard and fast rule, but it is a good indicator. Returning to historical foundations for a moment, many excellent healers did not accept money for their "gifts." They considered their work a kind of divine calling, for which some food, a beverage, or a service could be exchanged. Edgar Cayce, at the turn of the century, was just such an individual.

Modern times have moved us away from the barter system, but I still believe it has merit, especially in metaphysical settings. Exchanging services for services and talents for talents is a far more equitable arrangement than trying to put a dollar value on health. Again, I must stress that not all good healers offer this flexibility, simply because there are those in every group who will abuse the system for a "freebie." In this instance, patients must exhibit as much honor and scruples as they expect from their healers!

Once you finally discover a healer with whom you feel comfortable and confident, continue to remain fully informed and involved in your treatment. Share the healer's name with other people in need, and remember to thank the healer for his or her gift to you. Healers are people too, and knowing that they've helped us is the greatest recompense that healers receive.

Be well.

BIBLIOGRAPHY

Ainsworth-Davis, James R. *Cooking through the Centuries*. London: Jim Dent & Sons, 1931.

Arnold, John P. *Origin & History of Beer & Brewing*. Chicago: Wahl-Henius Institute of Fermentology, 1911.

Baer, Randall N. and Vicki V. *The Crystal Connection*. San Francisco: Harper & Row, 1986.

Baginski, Bodo. *Reiki*. Los Angeles: Life Rhythm Publications, 1988.

Baker, Jeannine Parvati. *Conscious Conception*. Berkeley, North Atlantic, 1986.

Baldwin, Rahima. *Special Delivery*. Berkeley: Celestial Arts, 1986.

Bartlett, John. *Familiar Quotations*. Boston: Little Brown & Company, 1938.

Benson, Herbert. *The Relaxation Response*. New York: Avon, 1976.

Bergson, Anika. *Zone Therapy*. New York: Winsor Publishing, 1974.

Beyerl, Paul. *Master Book of Herbalism*. Custer, WA: Phoenix Publishing, 1984.

Birren, Faber. *Color Psychology and Color Therapy*. Secaucus, NJ: Citadel Press, 1950.

Black, William George. *Folk Medicine*. New York: Burt Franklin, 1883.

Blate, Michael. *The Natural Healer's Acupressure Handbook*. Ft. Lauderdale, FL: Falkynor Books, 1983.

Borysenko, Joan. *Minding Our Bodies, Mending the Mind*. Reading, MA: Addison-Wesley, 1987.

Bravo, Brett. *Crystal Healing Secrets*. New York: Warner Books, 1988.

Brennan, Barbara Ann. *Hands of Light*. New York: Bantam, 1988.

Brody, Jane. *Jane Brody's Nutrition Book*. New York: Bantam, 1987.

Browne, Lewis. *The Believing World*. New York: Macmillan Company, 1959.

Budge, E. A. Wallis. *Amulets & Superstitions*. New York: Dover Publications, 1978.

Capra, Fritof. *The Tao of Physics*. New York: Bantam, 1977.

Cavendish, Richard. *History of Magic*. New York: Taplinger, 1977.

———. ed. *Man, Myth & Magic*. London: Purnell, 1972.

Chase, A. W. *Information for Everybody*. Ann Arbor, MI: R.A. Beal, 1870.

Chocron, Daya Sari. *Healing with Crystals & Gemstones.* York Beach, ME: Samuel Weiser, 1983.

Clark, Linda A. *The Ancient Art of Color Therapy.* Old Grenwich, CT: Devin Adair Co., 1975.

Clarkson, Rosetta. *Green Enchantment.* New York: Mcmillian Publishing, 1940.

Cohen, Sherry Suib. *The Magic of Touch.* New York: HarperCollins, 1987.

Cole, Dr. Raymond. *Wellpower.* River Rouge, MI: Wellpower Publications, 1984.

Conway, D. J. *Ancient Shining Ones.* St. Paul, MN: Llewellyn Publications, 1993.

Cristiani, R. S. *Treatise on Perfumery.* London: Baird & Co., 1877.

Crowley, Brian and Ester. *Words of Power: Sacred Sounds of East and West.* St. Paul, MN: Llewellyn, 1991.

Cummings, Charles. *Eco-Spirituality.* New York: Paulist Press, 1991.

Cummings, Stephen. *Homeopathic Medicines.* Los Angeles: J. P. Tarcher, 1991.

Cunningham, Scott. *Earth, Air, Fire & Water.* St. Paul, MN: Llewellyn, 1991.

———. *The Magic in Food.* St. Paul, MN: Llewellyn, 1991.

Davis, Elizabeth. *Heart & Hands: A Midwife's Guide to Pregnancy and Birth.* Berkeley: Celestial Arts, 1987.

Davison, Michael Worth, ed. *Everyday Life Through the Ages.* London: Reader's Digest, 1992.

Drury, Nevill. *Dictionary of Mysticism & the Occult.* New York: HarperCollins, 1985.

Ehrenreich, Barbara and Deirdre English. *Witches, Midwives & Nurses: A History of Women Healers.* New York: Feminist Press, 1973.

Farrar, Janet and Stewart. *The Witches God.* Custer, WA: Phoenix Publishing, 1989.

———. *The Witches Goddess.* Custer, WA: Phoenix Publishing, 1987.

Felding, William J. *Strange Superstitions & Magical Practices.* New York: Paperback Library, 1968.

Fleck, Henrietta. *Introduction to Nutrition.* 4th ed. New York: Macmillian Publishing, 1981.

Ford, Dr. Clyde W. *Compassionate Touch.* New York: Simon & Schuster, 1993.

Fox, William. *The Working Man's Model Family Botanic Guide*, 1907. Reprint: Mokelumne, CA: Mokelumne, 1963.

Gardner, Joy. *Healing Yourself During Pregnancy*. Freedom, CA: Crossing Press, 1987.

Garfield, Laeh Maggie. *Sound Medicine*. Berkeley, CA: Celestial Arts, 1987.

Garudas. *Flower Essences and Vibrational Healing*. San Rafael, CA: Cassandra Press, 1983.

Gaskin, Ina May. *Spiritual Midwifery*. Summertown, TN: Book Publishing Co.

Gerber, Dr. Richard. *Vibrational Medicine*. Santa Fe, NM: Bear & Co., 1988.

Gimbel, Theo. *Healing with Color and Light*. New York: Fireside Books, 1994.

Gordon, Leslie. *Green Magic*. New York: Viking Press, 1977.

Green, Julien. *God's Fool: The Life and Times of St. Francis of Assisi*. San Francisco: HarperSanFrancisco, 1985.

Grof, Stanislav. *The Adventure of Self Discovery*. Albany, NY: State University of New York Press, 1988.

Gutmanis, June. *Kahuna La'au Lapa'au*. Aiea, HI: Island Heritage Books, 1976.

Haggard, Howard W. *Mystery, Magic & Medicine*. Garden City, NY: Doubleday Doran, 1933.

Hall, Manly Palmer. *Secret Teachings of All Ages*. Los Angeles: Philosophical Research Society, 1977.

Hardin, Jesse. *The Kokopelli Seed*. Reserve, NM: Earthen Spirituality Project, n.d.

———. *Oikos: Songs for the Living Earth* (tape). Reserve, NM: Earthen Spirituality Project, n.d.

———. *Totem: Animal Teachers and the ReWilding of Humanity*. Reserve, NM: Earthen Spirituality Project, n.d.

Harlan, William. *Illustrated History of Eating & Drinking through the Ages*. New York: American Heritage Publishers, 1968.

Hoffmann, David. *Herbalism*. Dorset, England: Element, 1991.

Hendricks, Rhoda. *Mythologies of the World*. New York: McGraw Hill, 1979.

Inglis, Brian and Ruth West. *The Alternative Health Guide*. New York: Alfred A. Knoph, 1983.

Jung, C. G. *The Portable Jung*. Joseph Campbell, ed. New York: Vintage, 1971.

Kastner, Mark. *Alternative Healing.* Los Angeles: Halcyon Publishing, 1993.

Kilner, Walter J. *The Human Aura.* Secaucus, NJ: Citadel Press, 1965.

Kitzinger, Sheila. *Homebirth.* New York: Dorling Kindersley, 1991.

Koehler, Nan. *Artemis Speaks: VBAC Stories & Natural Childbirth Information.* Occidental, CA: Jerald Brown, 1985.

Krieger, Dolores. *The Therapueutic Touch.* New York: Fireside, 1979.

Kunz, George F. *Curious Lore of Precious Stones.* New York: Dover Publications, 1913.

Kushi, Michio. *The Book of Macrobiotics: The Universal Way of Health and Happiness.* Tokyo: Japan Publications, 1977.

Lawrence, D. Baloti and Lewis Harrison. *Massageworks.* New York: Perigee Books, 1983.

Leach, Maria, ed. *Funk & Wagnall's Standard Dictionary of Folklore, Mythology and Legend,* New York: HarperCollins, 1972.

Leboyer, Frederick. *Birth Without Violence.* New York: Knopf, 1975.

Loewe, Michael, and Carmen Blacker, eds. *Oracles & Divination.* Boston: Shambhala, 1981.

Lone Wolf Circles (Jesse Hardin). *Full Circle: A Song of Earthen Spirituality.* St. Paul, MN: Llewellyn, 1991.

Long, Carolyn K. "Reflexology" in *Massage Magazine,* Issue 59.

Lopez, Sonia, M.D. *Acupuncture.* New York: Harmony Books, 1988.

Lorrie, Peter. *Superstition.* London: Labyrinth, 1992.

Mariechild, Diane. *Mother Wit.* Freedom, CA: Crossing Press, 1988.

McCollum, Elmer V. *History of Nutrition.* Boston: Houghton Mifflin, 1957.

Metcalfe, Joannah. *Herbs & Aromatherapy.* London: Bloomsbury Books, 1993

Moody, Raymond A. *Coming Back.* New York: Bantam, 1990.

Monihan, Patricia. *Book of Goddesses & Heroines.* St. Paul, MN: Llewellyn Publications, 1993.

Murray, Michael T. *The Healing Power of Herbs.* Rocklin, CA: Prima Publishing, 1992.

Newall, Venetia. *Witchcraft & Magic.* London: Hamlyn, 1974.

Oesterly, W. O. E. *The Sacred Dance.* Cambridge MA: Cambridge University Press, 1923.

Opie, Iona and Moira Tatem. *Dictionary of Superstition.* New York: Oxford University Press, 1989.

Osborne, Duffield. *Engraved Stones.* New York, 1912.

Ostrander, Sheila and Lynn Schroeder. *Handbook of Psychic Discoveries.* New York: Berkley Medallian Books, 1974.

Ostrom, Joseph. *You and Your Aura.* London: Aquarian Press, 1987.

Regenstein, Lewis G. *Replenish the Earth.* New York: Crossroad, 1991.

Renfrew: Mary, et al. *Breastfeeding.* Berkeley: Celestial Arts, 1989.

Robbins, Andrew. *Diet for a New America.* Walpole, NH: Stillpoint, 1987.

Rodales Complete Illustrated Encyclopedia of Herbs. Claire Kowalchik and William Hylton, eds. Emmaus, PA: Rodale, 1987.

Rosato, Frank. *Fitness & Wellness.* St. Paul, MN: West Publishing, 1986.

Sargent, Denny. *Global Ritualism.* St. Paul, MN: Llewellyn, 1994.

Scheffer, Mechthild. *Bach Flower Therapy.* Rochester, VT: Inner Traditions, 1981.

Scott, Rev. J. Loughran. *Bulfinch's Age of Fable.* Philadelphia: David McKay, 1898.

Sharma, Dr. C. H. *Homeopathy & Natural Medicine.* London: Thorsons, 1975.

Siegal, Bernie. *Love, Medicine and Miracles.* New York: HarperCollins, 1990.

Singer, Charles. *From Magic to Science.* New York: Dover Publications, 1958.

Skinner, Charles M. *Myths and Legends of Flowers, Trees, Fruits & Plants.* Philadelphia: Lippincott, 1925.

Spence, Lewis. *Encyclopedia of Occultism.* New York: Fireside/Simon & Schuster, 1989.

Stark, Marcia. *Natural Healing.* St. Paul, MN: Llewellyn Publications, 1991.

Stein, Dianne. *Woman's Book of Healing.* St. Paul, MN: Llewellyn Publications, 1987.

Stephenson, Dr. James H. *A Doctor's Guide to Helping Yourself with Homeopathic Remedies.* New York: Parker Publishing, 1976.

Summer Rain, Mary. *Earthway.* New York: Pocket Books, 1990.

Tappan, Francis. *Healing Massage Techniques.* E. Norwalk, CT: Appleton & Lange, 1988.

Tannahill, Reay. *Food in History.* New York: Stein & Day, 1973.

Teeguarden, Iona Marsaa. *The Joy of Feeling.* Briarcliff Manor, NY: Japan Publications, 1987.

Telesco, Patricia. *Folkways.* St. Paul, MN: Llewellyn Publications, 1994.

―――. *Kitchen Witch's Cookbook.* St. Paul, MN: Llewellyn Publications, 1994.

Time-Life Editors. *Earth Energies.* Mysteries of the Unknown Series. Alexandria, VA: Time-Life Books, 1991.

―――. *Powers of Healing.* Mysteries of the Unknown Series. Alexandria, VA: Time-Life Books, 1989.

―――. *Witches & Witchcraft.* Mysteries of the Unknown Series. Alexandria, VA: Time-Life Books, 1993.

Thoreau, Henry David. *Walden.* New York: Vintage/Random, 1991.

Tisserand, Robert B. *The Art of Aromatherapy.* Rochester, VT: Healing Arts Press, 1977.

Tuleja, Tad. *Curious Customs.* New York: Harmony Books, 1987.

Ullmann, Dana. *Everybody's Guide to Homeopathic Medicine.* Los Angeles: J. P. Tarcher, 1984.

―――. *Homeopathy: Medicine for the 21st Century.* Berkeley, CA: North Atlantic Books, 1988.

Vithoulkas, George. *The Science of Homeopathy.* Athens: Athenian School of Homeopathic Medicine, 1978.

Walker, Barbara. *Womens Dictionary of Symbols & Sacred Objects.* San Francisco: HarperSanFrancisco, 1988.

Weed, Susan. *Wise Woman's Herbal for the Childbearing Year.* Woodstock, NY: Ash Tree, 1986.

Weiss, Brain L. *Through Time into Healing.* New York: Simon & Schuster, 1992.

Wilbur, Ken. *The Holographic Paradigm and Other Paradoxes.* Boston: Shambhala, 1985.

Williams, Judith. *Judes Home Herbal.* St. Paul, MN: Llewellyn Publications, 1992.

Woodhead, Henry, ed. *The American Indians.* Alexandria, VA: Time-Life Books, 1993.

Worwood, Valerie Ann. *Complete Book of Essential Oils & Aromatherapy.* San Rafael, CA: New World Library, 1991.

Zolar. *Encyclopedia of Ancient and Forbidden Knowledge.* New York: Fireside/Simon & Schuster, 1989.

INDEX

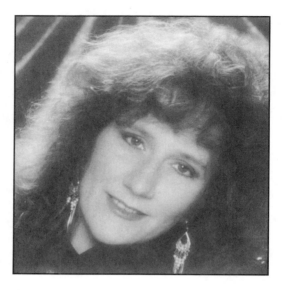

Patricia Telesco is a lifetime resident of western New York where she lives with her husband, children, and several well-loved pets. She has written 17 books, with more underway. Recent titles include *Seasons of the Sun* (Weiser, 1996), *The Sacred Stone Oracles* (Blue Pearl/Lotus Light, 1997), and *The Language of Dreams* (Crossing Press, 1997). She is a regular contributor to a variety of magazines and journals, including *Green Egg, Fate, New Moon Rising,* and *Four Winds Journal.* Telesco travels extensively, attending festivals and conducting lectures, workshops, and book signings at various bookstores around the country. She is also an ordained minister who actively supports religious freedom and understanding among different faiths, believing the bridge to a peaceful, enlightened future will be built with tolerance and respect.